EXERCISES IN ORAL RADIOGRAPHY TECHNIQUES
A LABORATORY MANUAL

Second Edition

Evelyn M. Thomson, BSDH, MS
Gene W. Hirschfeld School of Dental Hygiene
Old Dominion University
Norfolk, Virginia

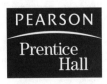

PEARSON
Prentice
Hall

Upper Saddle River, New Jersey 07458

Publisher: Julie Levin Alexander
Assistant to Publisher: Regina Bruno
Executive Editor: Mark Cohen
Associate Editor: Melissa Kerian
Editorial Assistant: Nicole Ragonese
Media Editor: John J. Jordan
Director of Production and Manufacturing: Bruce Johnson
Managing Production Editor: Patrick Walsh
Production Liaison: Christina Zingone
Production Editor: Jessica Balch, Pine Tree Composition
Manufacturing Manager: Ilene Sanford
Manufacturing Buyer: Pat Brown
Design Director: Cheryl Asherman
Design Coordinator/Cover Designer: Christopher Weigand
Director of Marketing: Karen Allman
Senior Marketing Manager: Harper Coles
Manager of Media Production: Amy Peltier
Media Project Manager: Stephen Hartner
Composition: Pine Tree Composition, Inc.
Printer/Binder: Command Web/Bind Rite
Cover Printer: Command Web/Bind Rite

Notice:
The author and the publisher of this volume have taken care that the information and technical recommendations contained herein are based on research and expert consultation, and are accurate and compatible with the standards generally accepted at the time of publication. Nevertheless, as new information becomes available, changes in clinical and technical practices become necessary. The reader is advised to carefully consult manufacturers' instructions and information material for all supplies and equipment before use, and to consult with a healthcare professional as necessary. This advice is especially important when using new supplies or equipment for clinical purposes. The author and publisher disclaim all responsibility for any liability, loss, injury, or damage incurred as a consequence, directly or indirectly, of the use and application of any of the contents of this volume.

Pearson Education Ltd., *London*
Pearson Education Australia Pty. Limited, *Sydney*
Pearson Education Singapore, Pte. Ltd.
Pearson Education North Asia Ltd., *Hong Kong*
Pearson Education Canada, Ltd., *Toronto*

Pearson Education—Japan, *Tokyo*
Pearson Educación de Mexico, S.A. de C.V.
Pearson Education Malaysia, Pte. Ltd.
Pearson Education, Upper Saddle River, New Jersey

PEARSON
Prentice
Hall

10 9 8 7 6 5 4 3 2 1
ISBN 0-13-171010-9

Contents

Preface

While dental hygiene and dental assisting students learn oral radiographic theory in the classroom, it is through laboratory practice that these students perfect the skills necessary to assume their professional roles. Currently textbooks are available for students to study oral radiology principles, but there remains a need for a laboratory manual that will challenge students to link theory with clinical practice. The purpose of this book is to provide dental hygiene and dental assisting students with concrete, practical exercises in oral radiographic procedures and interpretation. Designed to compliment basic oral radiology theory textbooks, *Exercises in Oral Radiography Techniques: A Laboratory Manual* serves as a workbook to guide the student in the practice of radiographic techniques.

It is the intent of this book to provide students and instructors with ready-made exercises, complete with directions for completing the activity; mounting diagrams to attach the finished radiographs; and pages that allow the student to turn in the assignments for instructor evaluation. Each of the student-driven activities requires minimal preparation by the instructor, and explicit directions guide the student in independent, self-paced practice.

USING THIS MANUAL

Each of the 15 exercises is easily adaptable for use in dental hygiene and dental assisting programs. The exercise modules may be used in any order, and are written in a style that allows the instructor to tailor the practice sessions to meet the needs of the program. For example, specific film-holding devices may be substituted for those suggested in the exercise. The inclusion of an "Instructor Demonstration" step at the beginning of each module provides an opportunity for the instructor to introduce products, procedures, and protocol which may be particular to that institution. Students may be directed to copy the mounting pages and continue practicing a technique until mastery, as determined by the instructor, is achieved.

Each exercise begins with an introduction, which provides an overview of the concepts, how the concepts relate to clinical practice, and the rationale for learning the material. Learning objectives are listed for each activity. To evaluate these objectives, study questions are included in each exercise module. Students are challenged to answer the questions based on the outcomes of the activity and/or from reading the material in the key-point outline. The outline following each activity serves as a convenient study guide to accompany a radiology theory textbook. This laboratory manual does not attempt to duplicate theory already covered in depth in most oral radiology textbooks. The intent of this manual is to compliment the basic theory text and be useful to the student as a study guide or as a review of the key concepts.

SUGGESTIONS FOR EDUCATORS

Although the exercises may be used in any order, the instructor may benefit from the sequencing explained here. Laboratory Exercise 1, which begins with a film processing and darkroom orientation activity, allows the student to begin the first week of the term or semester with a hands-on laboratory activity, while still receiving the necessary classroom instruction prior to safe operation of dental x-ray equipment. Laboratory Exercise 2 introduces the student to intraoral radiographic techniques with bitewing radiographs, followed by the periapical radiographic technique introduced in Laboratory Exercises 3 and 4. Paralleling, the technique of choice for quality imaging, is introduced in Laboratory Exercise 3. Laboratory Exercise 4 allows the student to gain a working knowledge of the bisecting technique, a skill often used to manage patients unable to tolerate the film packet placement required for the paralleling technique. Laboratory Exercise 5 builds on these basic techniques by helping the student to apply knowledge gained to utilize various commercially available film-holding devices.

Infection control protocol for radiographic services is formally introduced in Laboratory Exercise 6. While an instructor may choose to implement this module earlier, placing this activity a few weeks into the term is beneficial in two ways. First, most students will have had the opportunity to learn and practice infection control basics, such as the use of protective barriers and hand washing, in the patient-care pre-clinical course and can now expand on this knowledge to apply infection control methods specifically to the radiographic procedure. Additionally, by this time in a typical semester, the pre-clinical student will have begun to practice instrumentation skills intraorally. When students have had experience maneuvering around the oral cavity, they tend to be more prepared to perform film placement procedures. The initial apprehension that sometimes occurs with the first student partner practice is eliminated, and the students can concentrate on adapting the radiographic technique skills learned on teaching manikins or skulls to a real-life situation. Laboratory Exercise 7 builds on the initial partner practice by introducing patient management skills required for an apprehensive patient and the patient with a hypersensitive gag reflex, as well as alterations in radiographic techniques required for management of patients with anatomical conditions that interfere with the radiographic technique.

While each of the laboratory exercises challenges students to develop the skills required for film mounting, it is in Laboratory Exercise 8 that the student learns to appreciate the role identification of anatomical landmarks plays in film mounting. At this point in a typical semester, many students have acquired a basic knowledge of head and neck anatomy that can be applied to learning how to identify the radiographic appearance of these structures. Laboratory Exercise 9 provides an opportunity for the student to manipulate various exposure variables and identify the effects on the radiographic image. Evaluating these effects sets the stage for Laboratory Exercise 10 where the student is challenged to identify radiographic errors. Identification and correction of common radiographic errors provide valuable justification for maintaining a quality assurance program, introduced in Laboratory Exercise 11. Following acquisition of these basic radiographic skills, Laboratory Exercise 12 provides an opportunity for students to practice the interpretation skills necessary for clinical practice. Supplemental, extraoral, and digital radiographic techniques are introduced in Laboratory Exercises 13, 14, and 15.

ABOUT THE SECOND EDITION

To provide students with the guided exercises necessary to obtain dental radiographic skills, while providing instructors of oral radiology with a resource for meaningful laboratory activities, continues to be the goal of this lab manual. Features added to this second edition that enhance achievement of these goals include a competency and evaluation section in each of the 15 exercise modules that prompt the student to critically assimilate the learning objectives. Changes were made to the organization of the materials needed section and the preparation steps for each exercise to improve the readability of the book. Updates to Laboratory Exercise 5, Radiographic Techniques with Supplemental Film Holders, reflect the use of popular film-holding devices currently in use. Changes made to Laboratory Exercise 7, Patient Management and Student Partner Practice, focus more on developing student ability to manage difficult patient situations. Since the first edition published in 2000, technological advances prompt the addition of an exercise on digital imaging. State-of-the-art, evidence-based practices since the publication of the first edition have been added and are reflected throughout the manual.

ACKNOWLEDGMENTS

Exercises in Oral Radiography Techniques: A Laboratory Manual represents a collection of teaching strategies developed over the years of teaching oral radiology to dental hygiene and dental assisting students and interacting with colleagues. This book would not have been possible, without the support and assistance of the students, faculty, and staff at Old Dominion University, Gene W. Hirschfeld School of Dental Hygiene.

A very special note of appreciation goes to my husband Hu Odom for his loving support and encouragement.

Evelyn M. Thomson

Reviewers

Roberta Albano, RDH, CDA, MEd
Professor, Dental Assisting
Springfield Technical Community College
Springfield, Massachusetts

Sheri Billetter, CDA, EFDA, BS, FADAA
Chairperson, Dental Assisting
Linn-Benton Community College
Albany, Oregon

Mary Emmons, RDH, MEd
Program Director, Dental Hygiene
Parkland College
Champaign, Illinois

Deborah A. Graeff, RDH, MS
Professor, Dental Hygiene
Erie Community College
Williamsville, New York

Connie Myers Kracher, MSD
Program Director, Dental Assisting
Associate Professor, Dental Education
Indiana University–Purdue University–Fort Wayne
Fort Wayne, Indiana

Betty Reynard, RDH, EdD
Program Director, Dental Hygiene
Lamar Institute of Technology
Beaumont, Texas

Jacki Selby, MEd
Instructor, Dental Hygiene
Normandale Community College
Bloomington, Minnesota

Lucy A. Zarbo, RDH, BS
Assistant Professor, Dental Hygiene
Erie Community College
Williamsville, New York

Radiographic Film Processing and Darkroom Design and Maintenance

INTRODUCTION

Producing diagnostic quality radiographs is important in providing optimal oral health care for the patient. Although careful attention to placement and exposure of radiographs is considered important, often the same careful attention is not given to procedures performed in the darkroom. Carelessness in the darkroom and insufficient knowledge of processing activities can adversely affect the quality of radiographs produced. Poorly processed radiographs may have to be retaken. Retaking radiographs increases patient radiation exposure; therefore, it is important that the dental radiographer develop a working knowledge of the effects darkroom procedures have on the resultant radiograph. (Identification and correction of common radiographic processing errors is investigated in Laboratory Exercise 10, Identifying and Correcting Radiographic Errors.)

The purpose of this laboratory exercise is to introduce the student to dental radiographic film processing and darkroom maintenance. Using pre-exposed dental radiographs, the student will gain experience in processing dental radiographs.

OBJECTIVES

Following completion of this lab activity, you will be able to:

1. Identify the components of an intraoral film packet and specify the function of each component.
2. Identify the components of developer solution and specify the function.
3. Identify the components of fixer solution and specify the function.
4. Demonstrate proficiency in automatic and manual film processing methods.

5. Distinguish the difference between an overdeveloped and an underdeveloped radiographic image.

6. Discuss the advantages and disadvantages of automatic and manual processing methods.

7. Identify the characteristics of an efficient darkroom.

MATERIALS

Darkroom

Automatic processor

Manual processing tanks and chemicals

Thermometer, timer, film racks, film dryer (if available)

Pre-exposed intraoral films

PREPARATION

1. Study the chapter outline to prepare for this laboratory exercise. An understanding of the material presented in the outline is required to complete this activity.

2. Instructor demonstration may enhance knowledge of the laboratory exercise.

LABORATORY ACTIVITIES

Part 1: Automatic Processing—Individual Activity

1. Obtain one of the pre-exposed films labeled "A" for AUTOMATIC.

2. Follow the steps for automatic processing explained in the outline.

Part 2: Manual Processing—Group Activity

1. Work in small groups. Each student obtains one pre-exposed film labeled "M" for MANUAL.

2. Follow the steps for manual processing explained in the outline. Use one film processing hanger per group. Each individual should place his/her own film on the group film hanger. Label the film hanger with group name.

Part 3: Experiment 1—Group Activity

1. Work in small groups. Each student obtains one pre-exposed film marked "E1" for EXPERIMENT 1.

2. Follow the steps for manual processing explained in the outline *EXCEPT REDUCE THE STANDARD DEVELOPING TIME BY ONE-HALF.* (For example, if the standard developing time based on

the developer temperature is 5 minutes, then use 2.5 minutes of developing time for this experiment.)

3. Continue standard manual processing procedure. (The rinse, fix, wash, and dry times are **NOT** altered.)

Part 4: Experiment 2—Group Activity

1. Work in small groups. Each student obtains one pre-exposed film marked "E2" for EXPERIMENT 2.

2. Follow the steps for manual processing *EXCEPT INCREASE THE STANDARD DEVELOPING TIME BY ONE-HALF.* (For example, if the standard developing time based on the developer temperature is 5 minutes, then use 7.5 minutes of developing time for this experiment.)

3. Continue standard manual processing procedure. (The rinse, fix, wash, and dry times are **NOT** altered.)

COMPETENCY AND EVALUATION

1. Mount the processed films on the simulated film mounts that follow. Secure with a piece of tape placed along the top edge of the film only, so that the films may be raised slightly to allow light underneath for ease of viewing. The use of removable transparent tape will allow the film mount page to be used more than once.

2. Examine each of the processed films. Compare the manually processed films, and observe any differences in the density (overall darkness or lightness) of the images.

3. Obtain instructor feedback. Identify whether the processing methods were performed correctly.

4. The film mount page may be copied if additional practice is required to achieve competency.

5. Repeat Part 1, Part 2, Part 3, and/or Part 4 at the direction of your instructor.

6. Compare the two processing methods discussed in this exercise. What did you discover to be advantages and disadvantages of each of the skills you learned by completing this exercise? Give examples of situations in which one method may be an advantage over the other.

7. Complete the study questions.

NAME _____

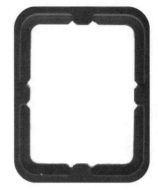

Part 1: Automatically Processed Film

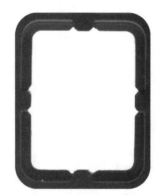

Part 2: Manually Processed Film (Standard): "M"

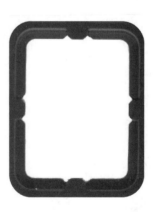

Part 3: Experiment 1: "E1"

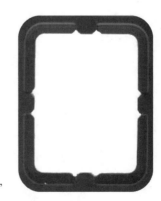

Part 4: Experiment 2: "E2"

Radiographic Film Processing and Darkroom Design and Maintenance **5**

I. Radiographic film
   A. Intraoral film packet components and function
      1. Film—image receptor (one or two films per packet)
      2. Outer plastic or paper wrap—moisture proof
      3. Black paper—light-tight
      4. Lead foil—absorbs scatter radiation
   B. Intraoral film composition
      1. Base—polyester plastic
      2. Adhesive
      3. Emulsion
         a. Silver halide crystals—light and x-ray sensitive component of the film
         b. Gelatin—suspends and evenly disperses the silver halide crystals
      4. Protective coating

II. Radiographic film processing
   A. Five basic processing steps
      1. Develop
         a. Hydroquinone—reducing agent
         b. Sodium carbonate—activator
         c. Potassium bromide—restrainer
         d. Sodium sulfite—preservative
         e. Distilled water—solvent
      2. Rinse
         a. Water
         b. Removes residual developer from film
      3. Fix
         a. Sodium thiosulfate—clearing agent
         b. Acetic acid—activator
         c. Potassium alum—hardening agent
         d. Sodium sulfite—preservative
         e. Distilled water—solvent
      4. Wash
         a. Water
         b. Removes all residual chemicals from film
      5. Dry
         a. Commercially made film dryer with heater and fan
         b. Air-dry method
   B. Processing methods
      1. Manual processing method
         a. Advantages
            1) Reliable (not subject to equipment malfunction)
            2) Easy standardization of quality
         b. Disadvantages
            1) Time consuming
            2) Requires manual regulation of solution temperature and manual timing methods
         c. Steps
            1) Select film hanger and label to identify films.

2) Open the light-tight cover of the manual processing tank, and stir the developer and fixer solutions to ensure even concentration throughout tank. (Use different stirring paddle for each, developer and fixer, to prevent contamination of solutions.)

3) Check developer temperature.

4) Refer to time/temperature recommendations of solution manufacturer, and set timer. (Optimal time/temperature for manually processed radiographs is 68 degrees F for 5 minutes.)

5) Lock darkroom door, turn off white light, turn on safe light.

6) Open film packets (recommended infection control procedure for opening film packets is discussed in detail in Laboratory Exercise 6, Infection Control and Student Partner Practice) and place films on hanger.

7) Immerse films into developer solution, and agitate film hanger for 5 seconds to release trapped air bubbles.

8) Set timer (time dependent on temperature of the developer solution).

9) Close light-tight cover while film is developing.

10) When the developing time is complete, under safelight conditions, open the light-tight cover and remove film hanger, with films attached, from developer solution.

11) Immerse film hanger into water rinse and agitate for 30 seconds.

12) Immerse film hanger into the fixer solution, and agitate film hanger for 5 seconds to release trapped air bubbles.

13) Activate timer for 10 minutes.

14) Close light-tight cover for the first 3 minutes of fixation. (It is safe to view the films under white light after 2 or 3 minutes of fixation for a "wet reading," following which the film must be returned to the fixer solution for completion of the 10 minutes of fixation time for archival quality films.)

15) Remove film hanger from fixer solution when time is up.

16) Immerse films in water wash for 20 minutes.

17) Place film hanger in a commercially made film dryer, or hang in the air-dry area when wash is complete.

18) Mount and label dried films.

2. Automatic processing method

  a. Advantages

    1) Increased volume of films may be processed in less time

    2) Automatic time/temperature standardization

  b. Disadvantages

    1) Possible equipment malfunction

    2) Initial unit expense

    3) Increased maintenance required for optimal output

    4) Increased chemical depletion

  c. Steps

    1) Turn on automatic processing unit.

2) Set appropriate time/temperature as indicated by the unit.
3) Lock darkroom door, turn off white light, turn on safe light.
4) Open film packets (recommended infection control procedure for opening film packets is discussed in detail in Laboratory Exercise 6, Infection Control and Student Partner Practice), and place films into automatic processor.
5) Allow rollers to take film before releasing.
6) Wait 10 seconds before placing an additional film into slot to avoid overlapping films.
7) Retrieve processed films when cycle is complete.
8) Mount and label dried films.

III. Processor maintenance (These recommendations are based on a typical private practice dental office use of approximately 30 intraoral films processed per day. In a larger clinical facility, where daily usage is much higher, these maintenance procedures should be performed more often.)

A. Manual processing maintenance
1. Daily
    a. Check solution levels for evaporation.
    b. Inspect underside of tank cover, clean, and wipe off condensation.
    c. Replenish developer and fixer solutions to maintain strength.
        1) Remove 6–8 ounces of developer (based on 1-gallon tank size), and discard in accordance with state and local agencies.
        2) Replace with fresh developer, filling tank.
        3) Remove 6–8 ounces of fixer (based on 1-gallon tank size), and discard in accordance with state and local agencies. (Because the fixer solution functions to remove the unexposed/undeveloped silver halide crystals, used fixer solution may contain silver ions in a concentration that prohibits disposing of this used fixer solution into the municipal sewer system in certain areas. A private contract waste removal service may be employed to dispose of used fixer in an environmentally safe way.) (Figure 1.1 ■)
        4) Replace with fresh fixer solution, filling tank.
    d. Inspect film hangers; they must be clean and dry.
    e. Check for proper solution temperature; adjust water flow as needed.
    f. Place cover over manual tanks overnight to prevent evaporation of chemicals.
    g. Shut off the running water and drain the rinse/wash tank at day's end.
    h. Inspect working area for cleanliness; wipe up chemical spills.
2. Weekly
    a. Check solution levels for evaporation.
    b. Perform quality assurance test to ensure correct strength of developing and fixing solutions. (See Laboratory Exercise 11, Radiographic Quality Assurance, for complete information regarding quality assurance tests for the darkroom.)
    c. Inspect rinse/wash water tank for calcium deposits.

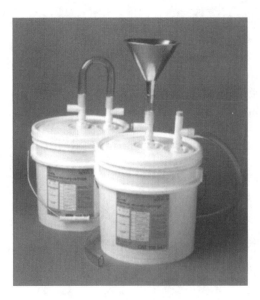

Figure 1.1 A commercial silver recovery system for use with automatic or manual processing system. (Reprinted from Publication D3-46, 1993, Courtesy of Eastman Kodak Company, Rochester, NY.)

   3. Monthly
      a. Empty the chemicals from the developer and fixer tanks, and discard in accordance with state and local agencies.
      b. Using a mild soap recommended by the manufacturer or plain water and a soft brush, clean and rinse the developer, fixer, and rinse/wash water tanks.
      c. Refill tanks with fresh chemistry.
      d. Maintain a quality assurance log, recording each monthly chemical change.
B. Automatic processor maintenance
   1. Daily
      a. Check solution levels for evaporation.
      b. If unit is equipped with automatic replenishing tanks, check to be sure replenisher bottles are full of fresh developer and fixer.
      c. If unit is not equipped with automatic replenishing tanks, then manually replenish developer and fixer solutions to maintain strength.
         1) Remove 6–8 ounces of developer (based on 1-gallon tank size), and discard in accordance with state and local agencies. (Figure 1.2 ■)
         2) Replace with fresh developer, filling tank.
         3) Remove 6–8 ounces of fixer (based on 1-gallon tank size), and discard in accordance with state and local agencies. (Figure 1.1)
         4) Replace with 6–8 ounces of fresh fixer solution.
      d. Inspect the outside of the processor for cleanliness; use a soft damp cloth to wipe any chemical spills and dust from the outside of the unit.
      e. Run a commercially made roller-transport cleaning sheet through the processor at the beginning of each day. This specially designed cleaning sheet will remove any debris from

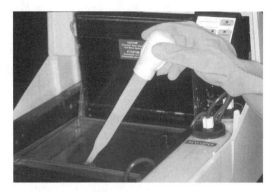

Figure 1.2 Removing 6–8 ounces of developer solution is easily achieved with a kitchen basting utensil.

the rollers, and roller movement will stir the solutions, readying them for processing patient films.

    f. Remove automatic processor cover overnight to prevent condensation that may form from dripping back down onto the rollers and contaminating them.

2. Weekly

    a. Remove roller-transports and use a clean, nonabrasive cleanser recommended by manufacturer or plain water and soft brush or sponge to thoroughly clean the rollers.

    b. Allow roller-transports to air dry overnight; in morning, rinse roller-transports with plain water and reassemble into unit.

3. Monthly

    a. Empty the chemicals from the developer and fixer tanks and discard in accordance with state and local agencies.

    b. Using a mild soap recommended by the manufacturer or plain water and a soft brush or sponge, clean and rinse the developer and fixer tanks.

    c. Refill tanks with fresh chemistry.

    d. Inspect the transport-rollers and gears for wear and/or damage and reassemble into unit.

    e. Using a thermometer, manually check the developer solution temperature to ensure proper temperature regulation by the unit.

    f. Maintain a quality assurance log, recording each monthly chemical change.

4. Periodically (as recommended by unit manufacturer)

    a. Remove the roller-transport system from the rinse/wash and dryer section of the unit, and clean and inspect for wear and/or damage.

    b. Inspect and lubricate the gear mechanism.

IV. Darkroom design

  A. Physical characteristics

    1. Light-tight

    2. Minimum of 16 square feet

    3. Located near patient treatment area

  B. Lighting

    1. Safe lighting

      a. Achieved through the use of an incandescent bulb shielded with a filter or a special LED (light emitting diode) bulb

b. Red filter or LED bulb safe for all types of film
c. Amber filter safe for "D" speed intraoral film only; not safe for use with "E" or "F" speed intraoral film; not safe for use with extroral film
d. 7½- to 15-watt incandescent bulb used with filter
e. Light must be positioned at least 4 feet from working area where films will be handled

2. White light
a. Room lighting for darkroom maintenance
b. View box lighting for wet readings

3. Other light
a. All other sources of light should be eliminated.
b. Blue/green indicator lights, such as those found on other equipment which may be kept in the darkroom should be eliminated or masked. (Figure 1.3 ■)
c. Luminous dials on watch faces or other equipment should not be used in the darkroom.

C. Plumbing
1. Temperature control for heating/cooling processing solutions
2. Deep utility sink, with goose-neck faucets for cleaning/maintenance of processing tanks
3. Sink for hand washing

D. Equipment
1. Necessary equipment
a. Processor tanks or automatic processing unit with solutions and means of replenishing those solutions
b. Thermometer
c. Timer

2. Supplemental equipment
a. Film dryer
b. Film duplicator unit
c. Film identification unit for extraoral radiographs
d. Cleaning supplies: tubs and brushes for cleaning automatic processor roller transports and manual solution tanks, container for used fixer waste or silver reclaiming unit, container to collect discarded lead foil from intraoral film packets for environmentally safe disposal or recycling
e. Infection control supplies: disinfectant, antimicrobial soap, gloves

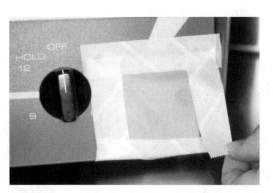

Figure 1.3 Placing a mask over a green indicator light on equipment located in the darkroom.

E. Documentation
   1. Record of processing solution maintenance and processor cleaning
   2. Patient film identification
   3. Chemical inventory
   4. Posted processing steps, equipment operation instructions, and recommended time/temperature processing charts

BIBLIOGRAPHY

Eastman Kodak Company. *Exposure and Processing for Dental Radiography.* Rochester, NY: Eastman Kodak Company; 1994.

Frommer, HH, Stabulas-Savage, JJ. *Radiology for the Dental Professional,* 8th ed. St. Louis: Elsevier Mosby; 2005: 118-145.

Thomson, EM. Developing an environmentally sound oral health practice. *Access;* 1996: 10:19–26.

1. Which of the following provides a moisture-resistant barrier for the film?
   A. Plastic/paper wrap
   B. Black paper
   C. Lead foil
   D. Gelatin

2. The light and x-ray–sensitive component of the film is the:
   A. Base
   B. Adhesive
   C. Emulsion
   D. Protective coating

3. The undeveloped and unexposed silver halide crystals are removed from the emulsion by:
   A. Acetic acid
   B. Hydroquinone
   C. Potassium alum
   D. Sodium thiosulfate
   E. Water

4. Exposed silver halide crystals are reduced to black metallic silver by:
   A. Acetic acid
   B. Hydroquinone
   C. Potassium alum
   D. Sodium thiosulfate
   E. Water

5. The optimum developing temperature for *manually* processing an intraoral film for 5 minutes would be:
   A. 48° F
   B. 58° F
   C. 68° F
   D. 78° F
   E. 88° F

6. Provided Parts 2, 3, and 4 of the laboratory activities were performed correctly, there should be a difference in density (overall darkness/lightness) between the manually processed standard film "M" and the EXPERIMENT 1 "E1" and EXPERIMENT 2 "E2" films. Compared with the standard film "M," which of the following films is lighter?
   A. "E1"
   B. "E2"

7. Provided Parts 2, 3, and 4 of the laboratory activities were performed correctly, there should be a difference in density (overall darkness/lightness) between the manually processed standard film "M" and the EXPERIMENT 1 "E1" and EXPERIMENT 2 "E2" films. Compared with the standard film "M," which of the following films is darker?
   A. "E1"
   B. "E2"

8. Overdevelopment will result in a
   A. Darker radiographic image
   B. Lighter radiographic image
9. Underdevelopment will result in a
   A. Darker radiographic image
   B. Lighter radiographic image
10. Dr. Perry A. Pical and Associates are moving to a new oral health care facility. Since it is the dental assistant's and dental hygienist's responsibility to reduce patient exposure by producing the highest quality radiographs, you have been called on to design and supply an efficient darkroom for the new practice setting. As you prepare plans for the new facility keep in mind the following:

    • What lighting/plumbing needs does your darkroom require?

    • What contents are essential for manual and automatic processing?

    • What type of record keeping is necessary? Why?

    • What role does location and size of the darkroom play?

    • What have you discovered during your lab experience to be qualities of a good darkroom? What problems existed? What would you change in planning for Dr. Pical?

_____

_____

_____

_____

_____

_____

_____

_____

_____

_____

_____

laboratory exercise 2

Bitewing Radiographic Technique

INTRODUCTION

Bitewing radiographs are probably the most frequently performed intra-oral dental radiographic technique. Utilizing a size #0, #1, #2, or #3 film, bitewing radiographs image the coronal portion of both the maxillary and the mandibular teeth, plus a portion of the surrounding interproximal alve-olar bone, and therefore are useful in imaging both caries (dental decay) and periodontal disease involvement. When exposing bitewing radiographs, the intraoral film packet has traditionally been placed in the mouth with the longer dimension positioned horizontally. In fact, the size #3 film is espe-cially designed for exposing horizontal bitewing radiographs. (Figure 2.1 ■) However, a vertical placement of a film packet has been found to be more useful when the focus of the bitewing radiograph is on the periodontium or root caries. (Figure 2.2 ■) Vertical bitewing radiographs increase the amount of information imaged in the vertical direction. In cases of mod-erately advanced periodontal disease, the full extent of alveolar bone re-sorption may not be fully imaged on the horizontally placed bitewing radiograph. Whether positioned horizontally or vertically, precise angula-tion and meticulous attention to technique is needed to ensure quality di-agnostic bitewing radiographs. Even seemingly minor errors can render a bitewing radiograph undiagnostic.

This laboratory exercise is designed to introduce the student to hori-zontal and vertical bitewing radiographic techniques. The seemingly complex principles of image geometry involved in exposing bitewing radiographs

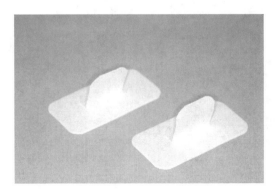

Figure 2.1 A size #3 film packet designed to be used to expose hor-izontal bitewing radiographs. Note the preattached tab.

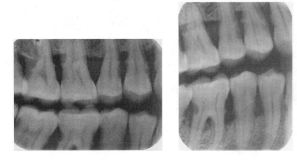

Figure 2.2 A comparison of the image achieved with a horizontally placed film packet (left) and a vertically placed film packet (right).

are organized into four basic steps. By simplifying the bitewing radiographic technique into four steps—packet placement, vertical angulation, horizontal angulation, and centering the x-ray beam—the student can easily produce and evaluate bitewing radiographs. Evaluation of the radiographic image is easier for the student when errors can be attributed to a specific step. Identification of which step caused the error allows the student to pinpoint which skill needs concentrated practice efforts. The simulated mount pages provided in this laboratory exercise may be copied to increase the amount of practice sessions the student requires to master the techniques.

There are a variety of commercially made film-holding devices on the market; however, this exercise uses the paper bitewing stick-on tab film holder. (Figure 2.3 ■) The use of this holder requires that the student develop the skills and ability to determine appropriate angles without relying on an external aiming device. Once the basic skills have been achieved, they can be carried over to other bitewing film-holding devices. (See Laboratory Exercise 5, Radiographic Techniques with Supplemental Film Holders.)

OBJECTIVES

Following completion of this lab activity, you will be able to:

1. Demonstrate proficiency in placing, exposing, and processing bitewing radiographs.

2. Correctly identify positive and negative vertical angulation of the PID (position indicating device)

3. Critique a bitewing series for correct (a) placement of the film packet intraorally; (b) vertical and (c) horizontal angulation of the PID; and (d) exposure of the film by centering the film packet within the x-ray beam.

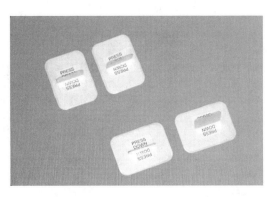

Figure 2.3 Paper bitewing stick-on tabs placed for vertical (top left) and horizontal (bottom right) bitewing radiographs.

MATERIALS

Teaching manikin or skull

Lead (or lead-equivalent) apron with thyroid collar

Size #1, #2, and #3 radiographic films

Bitewing film-holding device (stick-on tab—paper or foam type)

View box

Tongue blades

PREPARATION

1. Study the chapter outline to prepare for this laboratory exercise. An understanding of the material presented in the outline is required to complete this activity.
2. Utilize Table 2.1 to assist you with completing the exercises. Instructor demonstration may enhance knowledge of the laboratory exercise.
3. Prepare radiology operatory. Set up teaching manikin or skull. Ensure that correct "patient" positioning is achieved, i.e., occlusal plane parallel to the floor, mid-sagittal plane perpendicular to the floor.
4. Place lead apron (or lead-equivalent barrier) and thyroid collar over the "patient."

LABORATORY EXERCISE ACTIVITIES

Part 1: Horizontal Bitewing

1. Obtain four size #2 radiographic film packets.
2. Place bitewing holders on film packets.
3. Check posted exposure settings for the dental x-ray unit and set for bitewing radiographs.
4. Place and expose the series of bitewing radiographs in the following order:

   1st   right premolar bitewing

   2nd   right molar bitewing

   3rd   left premolar bitewing

   4th   left molar bitewing

   Note: Left-handed radiographers may use this order:

   1st   left premolar bitewing

   2nd   left molar bitewing

   3rd   right premolar bitewing

   4th   right molar bitewing

5. Process the four films.

TABLE 2.1 Film Packet Placement, Vertical and Horizontal Angulation, and Centering for Bitewing Radiographs for Adult Patients

Bitewing Radiograph	Film Packet Placement	Vertical Angulation	Horizontal Angulation	Centering (Direct the central ray of x-ray beam to this point of entry)
Central-lateral incisors Film size #1 or size #2 (vertical position)	Center the film packet to line up behind the right and left central and lateral incisors	+10	Direct the central rays perpendicularly through the left and right central incisor embrasure	A spot on the incisal plane between the maxillary and mandibular central incisors.
Canine Film size #1 or size #2 (vertical position)	Center the film packet to line up behind the canine; include the distal half of the lateral incisor and the mesial half of the first premolar	+10	Direct the central rays perpendicularly at the center of the canine	A spot on the incisal plane between the maxillary and mandibular canines.
Premolar Film size #2 (horizontal or vertical position)	Align the anterior edge of the film packet to line up behind the distal half of the maxillary or the mandibular canine; select the most mesially located canine	+10	Direct the central rays perpendicularly through the first and second premolar embrasure	A spot on the occlusal plane between the maxillary and mandibular second premolars.
Molar Film size #2 (horizontal or vertical position)	Align the anterior edge of the film packet to line up behind the distal half of the maxillary or the mandibular second premolar; select the most mesially located premolar	+10	Direct the central rays perpendicularly through the first and second molar embrasure	A spot on the occlusal plane between the maxillary and mandibular first molars.
Premolar-Molar Film size #3 (horizontal position)	Align the anterior edge of film packet to line up behind the distal half of the maxillary or the mandibular canine; select the most mesially located canine	+10	Direct the central rays perpendicularly through the second premolar and first molar embrasure	A spot on the occlusal plane between the maxillary and mandibular second premolars and the maxillary and mandibular first molars.

Modifid from *Essentials of Dental Radiography for Dental Assistants and Hygienists*, 8th ed. by O.N. Johnson and E.M. Thomson, Upper Saddle River, NJ: Prentice Hall, 2007: 192.

Part 2: Horizontal Bitewing Utilizing a Size #3 Film

1. Obtain two size #3 radiographic film packets.
2. If not already preattached by the manufacturer, place selected bitewing holders on film packets. (Figure 2.1)
3. Check posted exposure settings for the dental x-ray unit and set for bitewing radiographs.
4. Place and expose the bitewing radiographs in the following order:

   1st   right premolar-molar bitewing

   2nd   left premolar-molar bitewing

   Note: Left-handed radiographers may use this order:

   1st   left premolar-molar bitewing

   2nd   right premolar-molar bitewing
5. Process the two films.

Part 3: Vertical Bitewing

1. Obtain four size #2 and three size #1 radiographic film packets.
2. Place selected bitewing holders on film packets.

   Note: Two stick-on tab holders (paper type) may be placed on the anterior bitewing film packets to aid in placement in the anterior region. (Figure 2.4 ■)
3. Check posted exposure settings for the dental x-ray unit and set for bitewing radiographs.
4. Place and expose the bitewing radiographs in the following order:

   1st   central-lateral incisors bitewing

   2nd   left canine bitewing

   3rd   right canine bitewing

   4th   right premolar bitewing

   5th   right molar bitewing

   6th   left premolar bitewing

   7th   left molar bitewing

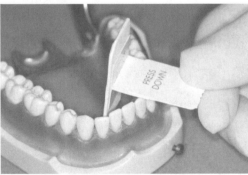

Figure 2.4 Using two stick-on tab bitewing film holders aids in film packet placement in the anterior region by extending the bite surface, allowing placement of the film packet well into the oral cavity where palatal height is greatest.

Note: Left-handed radiographers may use this order:

1st	central-lateral incisors bitewing
2nd	right canine bitewing
3rd	left canine bitewing
4th	left premolar bitewing
5th	left molar bitewing
6th	right premolar bitewing
7th	right molar bitewing

5. Process the seven films.

COMPETENCY AND EVALUATION

1. Mount the processed films on the simulated film mounts that follow. Secure with a piece of tape placed along the top edge of the film only, so that the films may be raised slightly, to allow light underneath for ease of viewing. The use of removable transparent tape will allow the film mount page to be used more than once.

   Note: Use the labial mounting method. (See Laboratory Exercise 8, Film Mounting and Radiographic Landmarks, for details.) The raised portion of the embossed dot is toward you (convex) when placing the film onto the page.

2. Place the page with the mounted films taped to it on a view box and evaluate for acceptability. Circle the ✓ where packet placement, vertical angulation, horizontal angulation, and centering were performed correctly, and the ✗ where performed incorrectly. Identify which error was made by placing an ✗ on the corresponding line.

3. Obtain instructor feedback. Identify which step (packet placement, vertical angulation, horizontal angulation, centering) needs improvement.

4. Repeat Part 1, Part 2, and/or Part 3 at the direction of your instructor. The film mount page may be copied to accommodate multiple practice attempts to achieve competency.

5. Compare the sets of bitewings with each other. Evaluate the images for diagnostic quality differences, and discuss which type (horizontal or vertical) and which size film produced the best images. Why? Assess your skills with each of the techniques. Did you find one or the other technique easier to place into position? Why? Discuss what type of oral conditions would be assessed for horizontal bitewings and for vertical bitewings. What did you discover to be advantages and disadvantages of each of the skills you learned by completing this exercise.

6. Complete the study questions.

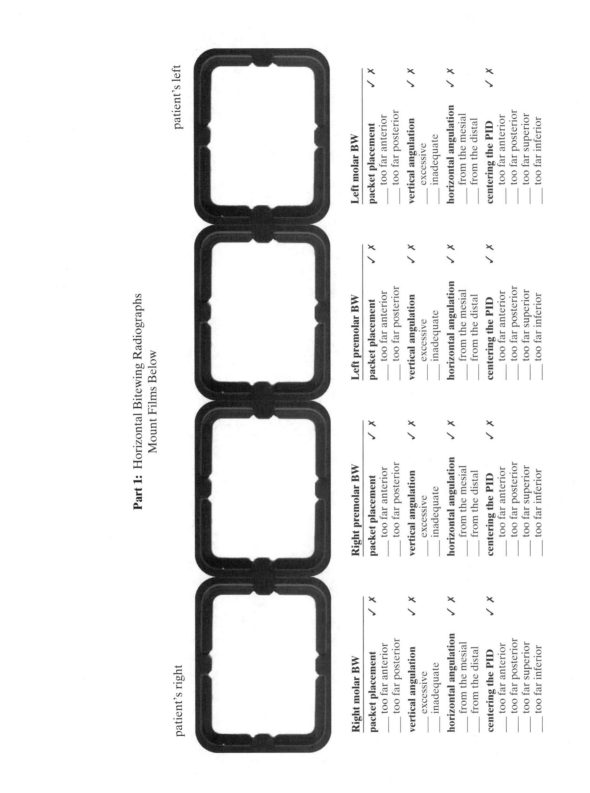

Part 1: Horizontal Bitewing Radiographs
Mount Films Below

patient's right

patient's left

Right molar BW

	✓	✗
packet placement		
___ too far anterior		
___ too far posterior		
vertical angulation	✓	✗
___ excessive		
___ inadequate		
horizontal angulation	✓	✗
___ from the mesial		
___ from the distal		
centering the PID	✓	✗
___ too far anterior		
___ too far posterior		
___ too far superior		
___ too far inferior		

Right premolar BW

	✓	✗
packet placement		
___ too far anterior		
___ too far posterior		
vertical angulation	✓	✗
___ excessive		
___ inadequate		
horizontal angulation	✓	✗
___ from the mesial		
___ from the distal		
centering the PID	✓	✗
___ too far anterior		
___ too far posterior		
___ too far superior		
___ too far inferior		

Left premolar BW

	✓	✗
packet placement		
___ too far anterior		
___ too far posterior		
vertical angulation	✓	✗
___ excessive		
___ inadequate		
horizontal angulation	✓	✗
___ from the mesial		
___ from the distal		
centering the PID	✓	✗
___ too far anterior		
___ too far posterior		
___ too far superior		
___ too far inferior		

Left molar BW

	✓	✗
packet placement		
___ too far anterior		
___ too far posterior		
vertical angulation	✓	✗
___ excessive		
___ inadequate		
horizontal angulation	✓	✗
___ from the mesial		
___ from the distal		
centering the PID	✓	✗
___ too far anterior		
___ too far posterior		
___ too far superior		
___ too far inferior		

Part 2: Horizontal Bitewing Radiographs—Utilizing a Size #3 Film
Mount Films Below

patient's right   patient's left

Right molar-premolar BW			**Left molar-premolar BW**		
packet placement	✓	✗	**packet placement**	✓	✗
___ too far anterior			___ too far anterior		
___ too far posterior			___ too far posterior		
vertical angulation	✓	✗	**vertical angulation**	✓	✗
___ excessive			___ excessive		
___ inadequate			___ inadequate		
horizontal angulation	✓	✗	**horizontal angulation**	✓	✗
___ from the mesial			___ from the mesial		
___ from the distal			___ from the distal		
centering the PID	✓	✗	**centering the PID**	✓	✗
___ too far anterior			___ too far anterior		
___ too far posterior			___ too far posterior		
___ too far superior			___ too far superior		
___ too far inferior			___ too far inferior		

patient's left

Part 3: Vertical Bitewing Radiographs
Mount Films Below

patient's right

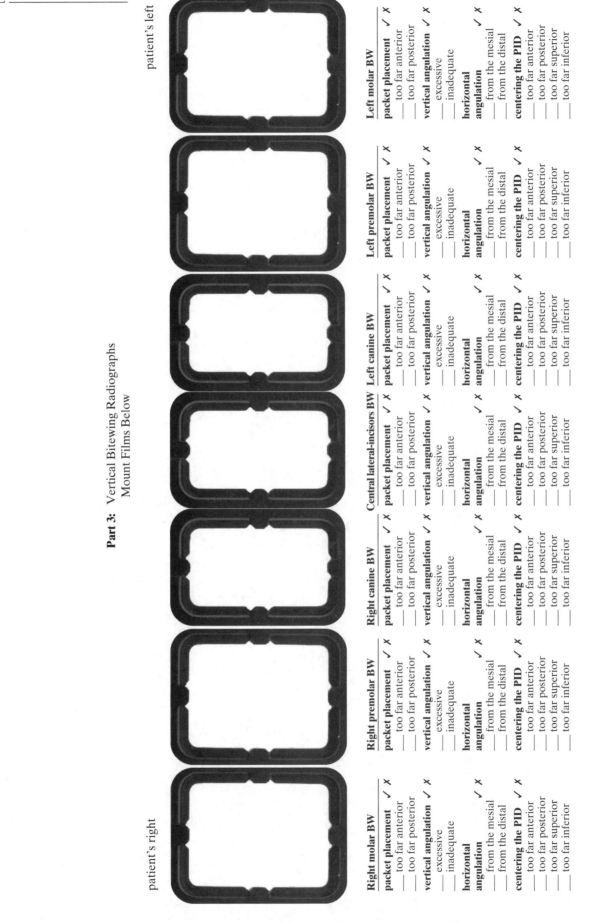

Right molar BW

packet placement ✓ ✗
___ too far anterior
___ too far posterior

vertical angulation ✓ ✗
___ excessive
___ inadequate

horizontal
angulation ✓ ✗
___ from the mesial
___ from the distal

centering the PID ✓ ✗
___ too far anterior
___ too far posterior
___ too far superior
___ too far inferior

Right premolar BW

packet placement ✓ ✗
___ too far anterior
___ too far posterior

vertical angulation ✓ ✗
___ excessive
___ inadequate

horizontal
angulation ✓ ✗
___ from the mesial
___ from the distal

centering the PID ✓ ✗
___ too far anterior
___ too far posterior
___ too far superior
___ too far inferior

Right canine BW

packet placement ✓ ✗
___ too far anterior
___ too far posterior

vertical angulation ✓ ✗
___ excessive
___ inadequate

horizontal
angulation ✓ ✗
___ from the mesial
___ from the distal

centering the PID ✓ ✗
___ too far anterior
___ too far posterior
___ too far superior
___ too far inferior

Central lateral-incisors BW

packet placement ✓ ✗
___ too far anterior
___ too far posterior

vertical angulation ✓ ✗
___ excessive
___ inadequate

horizontal
angulation ✓ ✗
___ from the mesial
___ from the distal

centering the PID ✓ ✗
___ too far anterior
___ too far posterior
___ too far superior
___ too far inferior

Left canine BW

packet placement ✓ ✗
___ too far anterior
___ too far posterior

vertical angulation ✓ ✗
___ excessive
___ inadequate

horizontal
angulation ✓ ✗
___ from the mesial
___ from the distal

centering the PID ✓ ✗
___ too far anterior
___ too far posterior
___ too far superior
___ too far inferior

Left premolar BW

packet placement ✓ ✗
___ too far anterior
___ too far posterior

vertical angulation ✓ ✗
___ excessive
___ inadequate

horizontal
angulation ✓ ✗
___ from the mesial
___ from the distal

centering the PID ✓ ✗
___ too far anterior
___ too far posterior
___ too far superior
___ too far inferior

Left molar BW

packet placement ✓ ✗
___ too far anterior
___ too far posterior

vertical angulation ✓ ✗
___ excessive
___ inadequate

horizontal
angulation ✓ ✗
___ from the mesial
___ from the distal

centering the PID ✓ ✗
___ too far anterior
___ too far posterior
___ too far superior
___ too far inferior

I. Bitewing radiographs
  A. Uses
    1. Image proximal surfaces
    2. Image intercrestal bone
    3. Caries detection
    4. Document periodontal status
    5. Image defective restorations
    6. Determine the presence of predisposing factors for periodontal disease: calculus, overhanging restorations
  B. Types
    1. Horizontal
      a. Film packet placed in the mouth with the long dimension positioned horizontally
      b. Considered the traditional bitewing film placement
    2. Vertical
      a. Film packet placed in the mouth with the long dimension positioned vertically
      b. Increased coverage of the teeth roots and the surrounding periodontium
      c. Particularly useful for imaging root caries and when bone resorption is extensive
      d. Often includes exposure of the anterior region
  C. Film sizes that can be used to expose bitewing radiographs
    1. Size #0
      a. Film size 22 mm × 35 mm recommended for children with primary dentition
      b. Short length of the film aids in placement of the film packet intraorally
      c. Suitable for primary dentition with minimal caries activity
      d. Height dimension of the film limits imaging pulp status when an extensive carious lesion is present
    2. Size #1
      a. Film size 24 mm × 40 mm recommended for children with primary dentition
      b. Longer length of the film may not be tolerated in a small oral cavity
      c. Longer length, if tolerated, will provide more diagnostic information
      d. Often used to expose vertical bitewings in the anterior region of adult patients
    3. Size #2
      a. Most common film size for exposing bitewing radiographs
      b. Suitable for children in transitional (mixed) dentition state and most all adults
      c. Film size 31 mm × 41 mm provides additional information about developing permanent teeth in the child patient
      d. Can be used to expose horizontal or vertical bitewings

4. Size #3
    a. Film size 27 mm $\times$ 54 mm specifically designed for the exposure of bitewing radiographs
    b. May not be used to expose vertical bitewing radiographs, especially if manufacture has pre-attached the bite tab in the horizontal position
    c. Longer length records all contact areas of one side of the oral cavity on one film
    d. Allows for the exposure of only two bitewing radiographs in a series: right premolar-molar and left premolar-molar
    e. Limited ability to clearly image all contacts because the premolar and molar areas of the oral cavity are not on the same horizontal plane
    f. Shorter height (only 27 mm compared with film size #2 which is 31 mm) may not be suitable for imaging interproximal alveolar bone, especially when bone loss is evident

D. Principal concepts
  1. White, unprinted side of the film packet positioned toward the teeth.
  2. Film is placed parallel to the facial surfaces of the maxillary and mandibular teeth of interest.
  3. Central ray of the x-ray beam is directed perpendicular to the film through the embrasures, between the teeth of interest.
  4. Film is held in place by a bite tab or other bitewing film-holding device.

II. Posterior bitewing radiographic procedure using size #2 film (horizontal or vertical film position)
A. Placement of the film packet
  1. Horizontal or vertical premolar bitewing radiograph
    a. Align the anterior edge of the film packet far enough forward to line up behind the middle of the maxillary or the mandibular canine; select the most mesially located canine.
    b. Ensure that the film packet is placed such that a portion of both the maxillary and mandibular canines, first and second premolars, and the mesial half of the first molars will be recorded on the film. (Figure 2.5 ■) (Vertical placement of the film packet may not be wide enough to record the first molars.)
    c. Place the film packet parallel to the facial surfaces of the premolars. (Figure 2.5)
  2. Horizontal or vertical molar bitewing radiograph
    a. Align the anterior edge of the film packet behind the middle of the maxillary or the mandibular second premolar; select the most mesially located second premolar.
    b. Ensure that the film packet is placed such that a portion of both the maxillary and mandibular second premolars, and first, second, and third molars (if erupted) will be recorded on the film. (Figure 2.6 ■) (Vertical placement of the film packet may not be wide enough to record the entire third molars. However, the most posterior interproximal contact should be imaged.
    c. Place the film packet parallel to the facial surfaces of the molars. (Figure 2.6)

 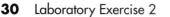

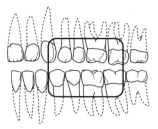

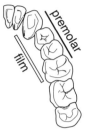

Figure 2.5 Film packet placement for horizontal premolar bitewing radiographs using a size #2 film. Note the line drawn to indicate that the film packet is positioned parallel to the facial surfaces of the premolar teeth.

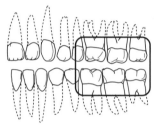

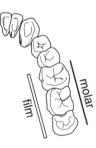

Figure 2.6 Film packet placement for horizontal molar bitewing radiographs using a size #2 film. Note the line drawn to indicate that the film packet is positioned parallel to the facial surfaces of the molar teeth.

B. Vertical angulation of the x-ray beam
   1. Determine the positive vertical angulation. Positive angulation is achieved by pointing the PID down toward the floor.
   2. Using the guide on the tube head, set the positive angulation to approximately +10 degrees for exposure of all posterior and anterior, horizontal and vertical bitewing radiographs on adult patients and to +5 degrees for bitewing radiographs on children who present with primary dentition. (Figure 2.7 ■) If no guide is present, vertical angulation is determined by using the floor as a reference point. When the PID is aligned parallel to the floor, the angulation is set at zero. When the PID is directed

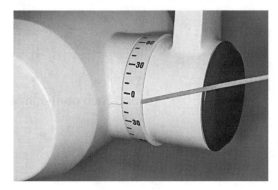

Figure 2.7 Using the guide on the tube head to determine +5 to +10 degrees vertical angulation.

perpendicular to the floor, the angulation is set at 90 degrees. To set the vertical angulation to +10 degrees, an estimation is made between these two easily identified points. (Figure 2.8 ■)

C. Horizontal angulation of the x-ray beam
   1. Determine the side-to-side placement of the PID.
   2. Align the PID such that the central ray of the x-ray beam will intersect the film perpendicularly. Perpendicular alignment of the beam can be achieved either of two ways:
      a. Direct the central ray of the x-ray beam through a predetermined interproximal space. (Figure 2.9 ■) Examine the

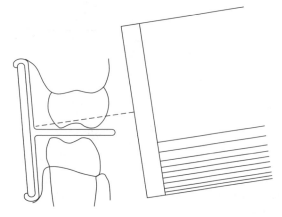

Figure 2.8 +5 to +10 degree vertical angulation utilized for bitewing radiographs.

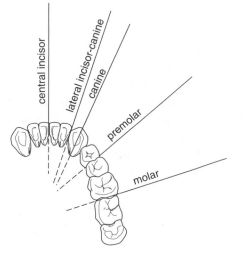

Figure 2.9 Horizontal angulation for bitewing radiographs when imaging the central incisors, central-lateral incisors, canine, premolar, and molar can be determined by directing the central ray of the x-ray beam between a predetermined interproximal space.

contact points of the patient's teeth to determine the correct angulation for aiming the central ray. Because of the larger size and rhomboidal shape of the maxillary posterior teeth, it is helpful to use the maxillary teeth when determining the correct horizontal angulation for bitewing radiographs.

    b. Using the open end of the PID as the reference point, align the PID such that the open end of the PID is parallel to the film in the horizontal plane. (Figure 2.10 ■) Visualizing the horizontal placement of the PID is easily achieved by placing a tongue blade or cotton-tipped applicator across the open end and rotating the tube head horizontally until the tongue blade or cotton-tipped applicator, and hence the open end of the PID, is parallel to the film. (Figure 2.11 ■)

  3. For a premolar horizontal or vertical bitewing radiograph, direct the central ray perpendicular to the film, between the first and second premolars. (Figure 2.9)

  4. For a molar horizontal or vertical bitewing radiograph, direct the central ray perpendicular to the film, between the first and second molars. (Figure 2.9)

D. Directing the x-ray beam over the film packet

  1. Determine the placement of the film packet.

  2. Using the bite tab film holder as a reference point, align the PID directly over the film packet. (Figure 2.12 ■) Correct placement of the PID can be achieved by placing the tongue blade as an extension of the PID. No part of the film packet should be visible beyond the diameter of the PID when extending the tongue blade. (Figure 2.13 ■)

  3. For a premolar horizontal or vertical bitewing, the central ray of the x-ray beam should be directed at a spot on the occlusal plane between the maxillary and the mandibular second premolars.

  4. For a molar horizontal or vertical bitewing, the central ray of the x-ray beam should be directed at a spot on the occlusal plane between the maxillary and the mandibular first molars.

III. Posterior bitewing radiographic procedure using size #3 film (horizontal position)

A. Placement of the film packet

  1. Premolar-molar bitewing radiograph

    a. Align the anterior edge of the film packet far enough forward to line up behind the middle of the maxillary or the mandibular canine; select the most mesially located canine.

    b. Ensure that the film packet is placed such that a portion of both the maxillary and mandibular canines, first and second premolars, and the first, second, and third molars will be recorded on the film. (Figure 2.14 ■)

    c. Place the film packet parallel to the facial surfaces of the second premolars and first molars. (Figure 2.14)

B. Vertical angulation of the x-ray beam

  1. Vertical angulation for bitewing radiographs utilizing a size #3 film is determined in the same manner as for posterior horizontal and vertical bitewings with a size #2 film.

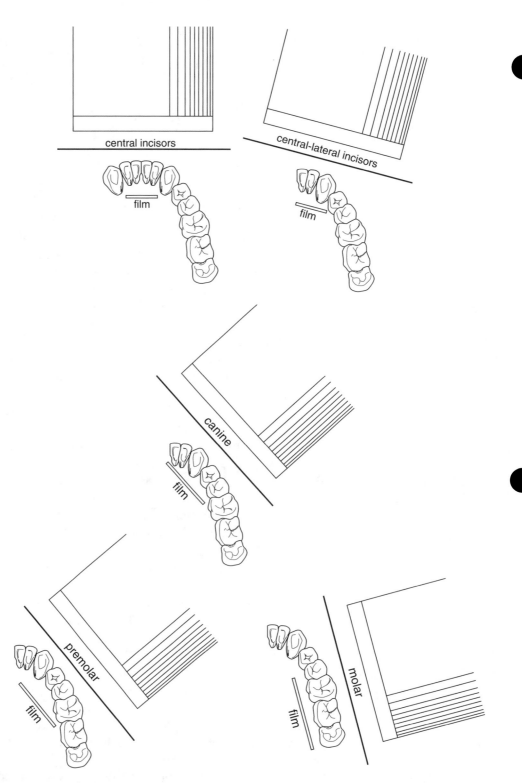

Figure 2.10 Horizontal angulation for bitewing radiographs when imaging the central incisors, central-lateral incisors, canine, premolar, and molar bitewing radiographs can be determined by aligning the open end of the PID parallel to the film packet. Note the line drawn to indicate that the open end of the PID is parallel to the facial surfaces of the teeth of interest. This line may be visualized through the use of a tongue blade.

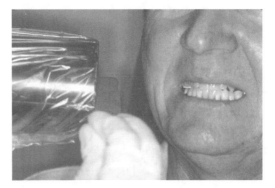

Figure 2.11 Using a tongue blade to visualize correct horizontal angulation.

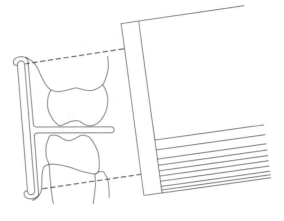

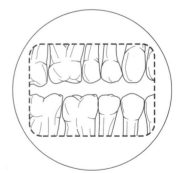

Figure 2.12 Film should be centered in the middle of the PID.

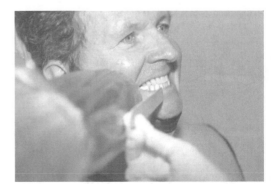

Figure 2.13 Using a tongue blade to visualize correct centering of the x-ray beam over the film packet.

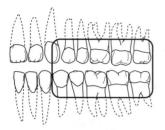

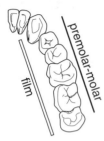

Figure 2.14 Film packet placement for horizontal premolar-molar bitewing radiographs using a size #3 film. Note the line drawn to indicate that the open end of the PID is parallel to the facial surfaces of the teeth of interest.

    2. Using the guide on the tube head, or the floor as the reference point, set the positive angulation to approximately +10 degrees. (Figure 2.8)

  C. Horizontal angulation of the x-ray beam

    1. Horizontal angulation for bitewing radiographs utilizing a size #3 film is determined in the same manner as for posterior horizontal and vertical bitewings with a size #2 film.

    2. Align the PID such that the central ray of the x-ray beam will intersect the film perpendicularly, through the embrasures of the teeth.

      a. For a premolar-molar bitewing radiograph utilizing a size #3 film, direct the central ray perpendicular to the film, between the second premolars and the first molars. (Figure 2.15 ■)

      b. Using the open end of the PID as the reference point, align the PID such that the open end of the PID is parallel to the film in the horizontal plane. (Figure 2.16 ■)

  D. Directing the x-ray beam over the film packet

    1. Directing the x-ray beam over the film packet utilizing a size #3 film is the same as for posterior horizontal and vertical bitewings with a size #2 film.

    2. Using the bite tab film holder as a reference point, align the PID directly over the film packet. (Figure 2.12)

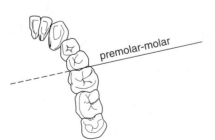

Figure 2.15 Horizontal angulation for premolar-molar bitewing radiographs utilizing a size #3 film can be determined by directing the central ray of the x-ray beam between the second premolars–first molars interproximal spaces.

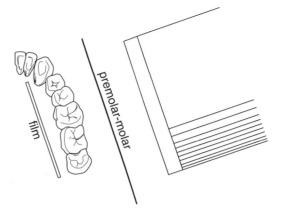

Figure 2.16 Horizontal angulation for premolar-molar bitewing radiograph utilizing a size #3 film can be determined by aligning the open end of the PID parallel to the film packet. Note the line drawn to indicate that the open end of the PID is parallel to the facial surfaces of the teeth of interest.

3. For a premolar-molar horizontal bitewing radiograph utilizing a size #3 film, the central ray of the x-ray beam should be directed at a spot on the occlusal plane between the maxillary and the mandibular teeth at the interproximal space between the second premolars and the first molars.

IV. Anterior bitewing radiographic procedure using size #1 film (vertical film position)

A. Placement of the film packet

1. Central-lateral incisors bitewing radiograph

a. Align the film packet behind the maxillary and mandibular left and right central incisors. Center these teeth on the film; include the mesial half of the maxillary and the mandibular lateral incisors. (Figure 2.17 ■)

b. Place the film packet parallel to the maxillary and mandibular central incisors. (Figure 2.17)

2. Canine bitewing radiograph

a. Align the film packet behind the maxillary and mandibular canines. Center the canines on the film; include the distal half

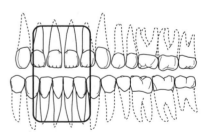

centrals

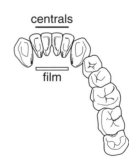

Figure 2.17 Film packet placement for central-lateral incisors vertical bitewing radiograph using a size #1 film. Note the line drawn to indicate that the open end of the PID is parallel to the facial surfaces of the teeth of interest.

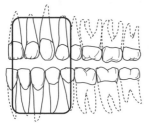

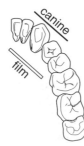

Figure 2.18 Film packet placement for canine vertical bitewing radiograph using a size #1 film. Note the line drawn to indicate that the open end of the PID is parallel to the facial surfaces of the teeth of interest.

of the maxillary and the mandibular lateral incisors and the mesial half of the maxillary and the mandibular first premolars. (Figure 2.18 ■)

    b. Place the film packet parallel to the maxillary and mandibular canines. (Figure 2.18)

B. Vertical angulation of the x-ray beam

    1. Vertical angulation for anterior vertical bitewing radiographs is determined in the same manner as for posterior horizontal and vertical bitewing radiographs.

    2. Using the guide on the tube head, or the floor as the reference point, set the positive angulation to approximately +10. (Figure 2.8)

C. Horizontal angulation of the x-ray beam

    1. Horizontal angulation for anterior vertical bitewing radiographs is determined in the same manner as for posterior horizontal and vertical bitewing radiographs.

    2. Align the PID such that the central ray of the x-ray beam will intersect the film perpendicularly, through the embrasures of teeth.

       a. For a central-lateral incisors bitewing radiograph, direct the central ray perpendicular to the film between the maxillary and mandibular left and right central incisors. (Figure 2.9)

       b. For a canine bitewing radiograph, direct the central ray perpendicular to the center of the maxillary and mandibular canines. (Figure 2.9)

       c. Using the open end of the PID as the reference point, align the PID such that the open end of the PID is parallel to the film in the horizontal plane. (Figure 2.10)

D. Directing the x-ray beam over the film packet

    1. Directing the x-ray beam over the film packet is determined in the same manner as for posterior horizontal and vertical bitewing radiographs.

2. Using the bite tab film holder as a reference point, align the PID directly over the film packet. (Figure 2.12.)
3. For a central-lateral incisors vertical bitewing, the central ray of the x-ray beam should be directed at a spot on the occlusal plane between the maxillary and the mandibular central incisors.
4. For a canine vertical bitewing, the central ray of the x-ray beam should be directed at a spot on the occlusal plane between the maxillary and the mandibular canines.

V. Errors
    A. Packet placement error
        1. Occurs when the film packet is not placed correctly intraorally
        2. Results in the appropriate teeth not being imaged on the film
        3. Packet placed too far anteriorly (Figure 2.19 ■)
        4. Packet placed too far posteriorly (Figure 2.20 ■)
    B. Vertical angulation error
        1. Occurs when the up and down angle of the PID is not set at +10 degrees when exposing bitewing radiographs on adults and +5 when exposing bitewing radiographs on children with primary dentition
        2. Results in unequal distribution of the arches on the resultant radiograph
        3. Excessive vertical angulation: angulation set greater than +10 degrees for adults and greater than +5 degrees for children (Figure 2.21 ■)
        4. Inadequate vertical angulation: angulation set less than +10 degrees for adults and less than +5 degrees for children (Figure 2.22 ■)
    C. Horizontal angulation error
        1. Occurs when the side-to-side angulation of the PID is not set such that the beam will intersect with the film perpendicularly

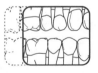

Figure 2.19 A horizontal molar bitewing radiograph demonstrating film packet placed too far anteriorly so as not to image the distal contact between the second and third molars.

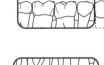

Figure 2.20 A horizontal premolar bitewing radiograph demonstrating film packet placed too far posteriorly so as not to image the contact between the canines and the first premolars.

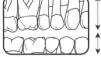

Figure 2.21 Excessive vertical angulation (greater than +10 degrees for an adult and greater than +5 degrees for a child with primary dentition) results in unequal distribution of the maxillary and mandibular arches, not imaging the alveolar bone on the mandible.

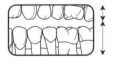

Figure 2.22 Inadequate vertical angulation (less than +10 degrees for an adult and less than +5 degrees for a child with primary dentition) results in unequal distribution of the maxillary and mandibular arches, not imaging the alveolar bone on the maxilla.

2. Results in superimposition of proximal surfaces of adjacent teeth (overlap error)
3. Occurs when the beam intersects with the film obliquely from the mesial direction (Figure 2.23 ■)
4. Occurs when the beam intersects with the film obliquely from the distal direction (Figure 2.24 ■)

D. Centering the x-ray beam over the film error
1. Occurs when the PID is not placed directly over the film packet
2. Results in an unexposed or clear area recorded on the film (cone-cut error)
3. Creates a cone-cut error when the beam is too far toward the anterior (Figure 2.25 ■)
4. Creates a cone-cut error when the beam is too far toward the posterior (Figure 2.26 ■)
5. Creates a cone-cut error when the beam is too far toward the superior (Figure 2.27 ■)
6. Creates a cone-cut error when the beam is too far toward the inferior (Figure 2.28 ■)

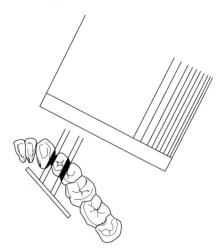

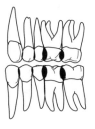

Figure 2.23 When the horizontal angulation intersects the film obliquely from the mesial, the most severe overlap occurs in the posterior region of the image.

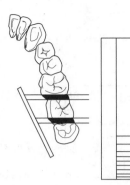

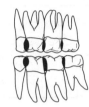

Figure 2.24 When the horizontal angulation intersects the film obliquely from the distal, the most severe overlap occurs in the anterior region of the image.

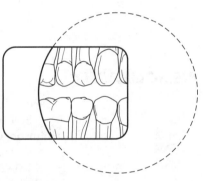

Figure 2.25 When the PID is not centered over the film, an unexposed or clear "cone-cut" area results. When the "cone-cut" is in the posterior region of the image, the PID was positioned too far anterior.

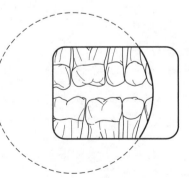

Figure 2.26 When the PID is not centered over the film, an unexposed or clear "cone-cut" area results. When the "cone-cut" is in the anterior region of the image, the PID was positioned too far posterior.

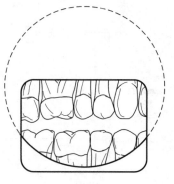

Figure 2.27 When the PID is not centered over the film, an unexposed or clear "cone-cut" area results. When the "cone-cut" is in the inferior section of the image, the PID was positioned too far superior.

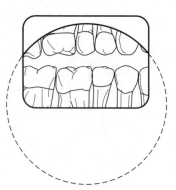

Figure 2.28 When the PID is not centered over the film, an unexposed or clear "cone-cut" area results. When the "cone-cut" is in the superior section of the image, the PID was positioned too far inferior.

BIBLIOGRAPHY

Haring, JI, Howerton, LJ. *Dental Radiography. Principles and Techniques,* 3rd ed. St. Louis, MO: Elsevier; 2006: 253–270.

Johnson, ON, Thomson, EM. *Essentials of Dental Radiography for Dental Assistants and Hygienists,* 8th ed. Upper Saddle River, NJ: Prentice Hall; 2007: 181–200.

Stabulas, JJ. Vertical bitewings: The other option. *Journal of Practical Hygiene;* 2002 11:46–47.

Thomson, EM. Dental radiographs for the child patient. *Dental Hygienist News;* 1993: 6:19–20, 24.

White, SC, Pharoah, MJ. *Oral Radiology Principles and Interpretation,* 5th ed. St. Louis, MO: Elsevier; 2004: 148–153.

1. Which of the following patients would benefit *most* from vertical bite-wing radiographs rather than horizontal bitewing radiographs?
   A. Age 5 years, primary dentition, slight gingival inflamma-tion, slight materia alba present
   B. Age 10 years, mixed dentition, moderate marginal and pap-illary gingivitis, moderate plaque present
   C. Age 25 years, permanent dentition, severe gingival inflam-mation, generalized probe readings of 5–8 mm
   D. Age 50 years, some missing teeth, generalized 1 mm reces-sion, probing depths range from 1 mm to 2 mm

2. Which of the following teeth should be imaged on a horizontal pre-molar bitewing?
   A. Distal portion of the central incisor, lateral incisor, canine, first premolar, mesial portion of the second premolar
   B. Distal portion of the lateral incisor, canine, first premolar, second premolar, mesial portion of the first molar
   C. Distal portion of the canine, first premolar, second premo-lar, first molar, mesial portion of the second molar
   D. Distal portion of the first premolar, second premolar, first molar, second molar, mesial portion of the third molar

3. Which of the following teeth should be imaged on a horizontal molar bitewing?
   A. Distal portion of the lateral incisor, canine, first premolar, second premolar, mesial portion of the first premolar
   B. Distal portion of the canine, first premolar, second premo-lar, first molar, mesial portion of the second molar
   C. Distal portion of the first premolar, second premolar, first molar, second molar, mesial portion of the third molar
   D. Distal portion of the second premolar, first molar, second molar, third molar

4. With *positive* vertical angulation, the PID (position indicating device) is pointing such that the x-ray beam will be directed:
   A. Up
   B. Down

5. With *negative* vertical angulation, the PID (position indicating device) is pointing such that the x-ray beam will be directed:
   A. Up
   B. Down

6. Which of the following is the correct vertical angulation for bitewing radiographs?
   A. −5 to −10 degrees
   B. −15 to −20 degrees
   C. +5 to +10 degrees
   D. +15 to +20 degrees

7. Through which interproximal space should the central ray of the x-ray beam be directed when exposing a *molar* bitewing radiograph?
   A. Between the canine and the first premolar
   B. Between the first premolar and the second premolar
   C. Between the second premolar and the first molar
   D. Between the first molar and the second molar
   E. Between the second molar and the third molar

8. Overlapped interproximal spaces results from an error made in which of the following?
   A. Packet placement
   B. Vertical angulation
   C. Horizontal angulation
   D. Centering the x-ray beam

9. Unequal distribution of the arches (i.e., seeing more of the maxillary arch and not enough of the mandibular arch) results from an error made in which of the following?
   A. Packet placement
   B. Vertical angulation
   C. Horizontal angulation
   D. Centering the x-ray beam

10. Cone-cut error results from incorrect
    A. Packet placement
    B. Vertical angulation
    C. Horizontal angulation
    D. Centering the x-ray beam

Periapical Radiographs— Paralleling Technique

INTRODUCTION

A dental radiographic examination plays an important role in identifying and diagnosing oral conditions. Periapical radiographs are particularly useful in that they image the entire tooth from incisal/occlusal edge to the tip of the tooth root. Diagnostic periapical radiographs should image at least 2 mm beyond the apex of the tooth to include information about the supporting bone, lamina dura, and periodontal ligament space. There are two radiographic techniques used to expose periapical radiographs, and the dental radiographer should develop skills necessary for both. However, the technique recommended by the American Dental Association and the American Academy of Oral and Maxillofacial Radiology for exposing periapical radiographs is the paralleling technique. Periapical radiographs taken utilizing the paralleling technique are more likely to be free of the image distortion typically found with the bisecting technique.

The same four basic steps—packet placement, vertical angulation, horizontal angulation, and centering the x-ray beam—that are utilized when placing and exposing bitewing radiographs (Laboratory Exercise 2, Bitewing Radiographic Technique) are employed when placing and exposing periapical radiographs. Learning the paralleling technique by following these four distinct steps will allow the student to consistently produce and evaluate periapical radiographs. Evaluation of the radiographic image is easier for the student when errors can be attributed to a specific step. Identification of which step caused the error allows the student to pinpoint which skill needs concentrated practice efforts. The simulated mount pages provided in this laboratory exercise may be copied to increase the amount of practice sessions the student requires to master the techniques. The use of removable transparent tape will allow the simulated mount pages to be used more than once.

There are a variety of commercially made film-holding devices on the market. This exercise uses the Stabe® (Dentsply Rinn) disposable, polystyrene bite block film holder (Figure 3.1 ■), but the student may be directed to complete the activity using the standard film-holding device at his/her institution. Many commercially available film-holding devices are designed with external aiming devices. These aiming devices are helpful

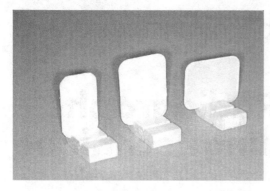

Figure 3.1 Stabe® disposable polystyrene film holder with size #1 and size #2 films placed vertically for anterior periapical radiographs and placed horizontally for posterior periapical radiographs.

aids in aligning the x-ray beam with the film, but the bulk and weight of the attachments may make the device difficult to position in the oral cavity on some patients. This may be true for children, adults with small or sensitive oral cavities or intrusive tori, or the patient with an exaggerated gag reflex. If the film holder is positioned incorrectly, the x-ray beam will be aligned inaccurately. The radiographer who can recognize accurate beam alignment without the use of an external aiming device may be better able to evaluate the position of the film regardless of the type of film holder used. A thorough understanding of film packet placement and vertical and horizontal beam angulation is needed to master the paralleling technique. This exercise uses a periapical film holder without an external aiming device, prompting the student to develop the skills and ability to determine appropriate angles. By creating this need to know correct angles and accurate image geometry, the student gains basic skills that may be carried over to any type of film holder. (See Laboratory Exercise 5, Radiographic Techniques with Supplemental Film Holders.)

OBJECTIVES

Following completion of this lab activity, you will be able to:

1. Demonstrate proficiency in placing, exposing, and processing anterior and posterior periapical radiographs using the paralleling technique.

2. Critique a full mouth series of intraoral radiographs consisting of anterior and posterior periapicals, for correct (a) placement of the film packet intraorally; (b) vertical and (c) horizontal angulation of the PID; and (d) exposure of the film by directing the x-ray beam over the film packet.

MATERIALS

Teaching manikin or skull

Lead (or lead-equivalent) apron with thyroid collar

Size #1 and size #2 radiographic films

Periapical film-holding device (disposable Stabe® film holders or similar device designed for use with the paralleling technique)

Viewbox

Tongue blades

PREPARATION

1. Study the chapter outline to prepare for this laboratory exercise. An understanding of the material presented in the outline is required to complete this activity.

2. Utilize Table 3.1 to assist you with completing the exercises. Instructor demonstration may enhance knowledge of the laboratory exercise.

3. Prepare radiology operatory. Set up teaching manikin or skull. Ensure that correct "patient" positioning is achieved. To image the maxilla, ensure that the maxillary occlusal plane is parallel to the floor; to image the mandible, ensure that the mandibular occlusal plane is parallel to the floor and the midsagittal plane must be perpendicular to the floor for both maxillary and mandibular exposures.

4. Place lead apron (or lead-equivalent barrier) and thyroid collar over the "patient."

5. The size and/or number of films included in a full mouth series of periapical radiographs varies among practices. The anterior periapical radiographic examination may include the exposure of 6, 7, or 8 periapical radiographs, whereas the posterior radiographic examination usually remains standard with the exposure of 8 periapical radiographs. (Figure 3.2 ■) This exercise will focus on the use of two of the most common full mouth series configurations: Figures 3.2A and 3.2B.

6. Obtain disposable Stabe® periapical film holders or similar device designed for use with the paralleling technique.

7. Orient the film packet in the film holder so that the embossed identification dot will be placed away from the apices of the teeth. Place the "dot in the slot" of the film holder to position the identification dot of the film packet toward the incisal/occlusal edges of the teeth. (Figure 3.3 ■)

8. Start with the anterior exposures. Beginning the examination with the more tolerable anterior film placements will help to gain the patient's confidence and cooperation with the procedure.

LABORATORY EXERCISE ACTIVITIES

Part 1: Periapical Radiographs Using the Paralleling Technique—Anterior Region

1. If using *Full Mouth Series A* for this exercise, you may choose to obtain six size #2 radiographic film packets; or six size #1 radiographic film packets; or a combination of five size #1 and one size #2 radiographic film packets. If using *Full Mouth Series B* for this exercise, obtain eight size #1 radiographic film packets.

2. Place film packet into the Stabe® film holder with the long dimension positioned vertically. (Figure 3.1)

3. Check posted exposure settings for the dental x-ray unit prior to placing each film packet, and set for the anterior region; adjust as needed for the maxilla and for the mandible, and for the canine and the central incisor regions.

TABLE 3.1 Film Packet Placement, Vertical and Horizontal Angulation, and Centering for Anterior and Posterior Periapical Radiographs for Adult Patients Utilizing the Paralleling Technique

Periapical Radiograph	Film Packet Placement	Vertical Angulation	Horizontal Angulation	Centering
Maxillary Central Incisors Use film size #1 or size #2	Center the film packet to line up behind the central and lateral incisors on both the right and left sides; if using a size #2 film, include the mesial halves of the canines.	Direct the central rays of the x-ray beam toward the film perpendicularly in the vertical dimension; the PID will be pointing down.	Direct the central rays of the x-ray beam perpendicularly through the left and right central incisor embrasure.	Center the film packet within the x-ray beam; direct the central rays of the x-ray beam toward the center of the film.
Maxillary Central-Lateral Incisors Use film size #1	Center the film packet to line up behind the central and lateral incisors on one side of the mouth; include a portion of the central incisor on the opposite side and a portion of the canine	Direct the central rays of the x-ray beam toward the film perpendicularly in the vertical dimension; the PID will be pointing down.	Direct the central rays of the x-ray beam perpendicularly through the central incisor and lateral incisor embrasure.	Center the film packet within the x-ray beam; direct the central rays of the x-ray beam toward the center of the film.
Maxillary Canine Use film size #1 or size #2	Center the film packet to line up behind the canine; include the distal half of the lateral incisor and the mesial half of the first premolar.	Direct the central rays of the x-ray beam toward the film perpendicularly in the vertical dimension; the PID will be pointing down.	Direct the central rays of the x-ray beam perpendicularly in the horizontal direction at the center of the canine.	Center the film packet within the x-ray beam; direct the central rays of the x-ray beam toward the center of the film.
Maxillary Premolar Use film size #2	Align the anterior edge of film packet to line up behind the distal half of the canine; include the first and second premolars, first molar, and mesial half of the second molar.	Direct the central rays of the x-ray beam toward the film perpendicularly in the vertical dimension; the PID will be pointing down.	Direct the central rays of the x-ray beam perpendicularly through the first and second premolar embrasure.	Center the film packet within the x-ray beam; direct the central rays of the x-ray beam toward the center of the film.
Maxillary Molar Use film size #2	Align the anterior edge of film packet to line up behind the distal half of the second premolar; include the first, second, and third molars.	Direct the central rays of the x-ray beam toward the film perpendicularly in the vertical dimension; the PID will be pointing down.	Direct the central rays of the x-ray beam perpendicularly through the first and second molar embrasure.	Center the film packet within the x-ray beam; direct the central rays of the x-ray beam toward the center of the film.

Mandibular Central Incisors Use film size #1 or size #2	Center the film packet to line up behind the central and lateral incisors; if using a size #2 film, include the mesial halves of the canines.	Direct the central rays of the x-ray beam toward the film perpendicularly in the vertical dimension; the PID will be pointing up.	Direct the central rays of the x-ray beam perpendicularly through the left and right central incisor embrasure.	Center the film packet within the x-ray beam; direct the central rays of the x-ray beam toward the center of the film.
Mandibular Central-Lateral Incisors Use film size #1	Center the film packet to line up behind the central and lateral incisors on one side of the mouth; include a portion of the central incisor on the opposite side and a portion of the canine.	Direct the central rays of the x-ray beam toward the film perpendicularly in the vertical dimension; the PID will be pointing up.	Direct the central rays of the x-ray beam perpendicularly through the central incisor and lateral incisor embrasure	Center the film packet within the x-ray beam; direct the central rays of the x-ray beam toward the center of the film.
Mandibular Canine Use film size #1 or size #2	Center the film packet to line up behind the canine; include the distal half of the lateral incisor and the mesial half of the first premolar.	Direct the central rays of the x-ray beam toward the film perpendicularly in the vertical dimension; the PID will be pointing up.	Direct the central rays of the x-ray beam perpendicularly in the horizontal direction at the center of the canine	Center the film packet within the x-ray beam; direct the central rays of the x-ray beam toward the center of the film.
Mandibular Premolar Use film size #2	Align the anterior edge of film packet to line up behind the distal half of the canine; include the first and second premolars and mesial half of the first molar.	Direct the central rays of the x-ray beam toward the film perpendicularly in the vertical dimension; the PID will be pointing up.	Direct the central rays of the x-ray beam perpendicularly through the first and second premolar embrasure.	Center the film packet within the x-ray beam; direct the central rays of the x-ray beam toward the center of the film.
Mandibular Molar Use film size #2	Align the anterior edge of film packet to line up behind the distal half of the second premolar; include the first, second, and third molars.	Direct the central rays of the x-ray beam toward the film perpendicularly in the vertical dimension; the PID will be pointing up.	Direct the central rays of the x-ray beam perpendicularly through the first and second molar embrasure	Center the film packet within the x-ray beam; direct the central rays of the x-ray beam toward the center of the film.

Modified from *Essentials of Dental Radiography for Dental Assistants and Hygienists*, 8th ed. by O. N. Johnson and E. M. Thomson, Upper Saddle River, NJ: Prentice Hall, 2007: 167–168.

A. 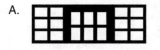 6 anterior periapical radiographs with size #2 film
8 posterior periapical radiographs with size #2 film
4 bitewing radiographs (horizontal or vertical) with size #2 film

B. 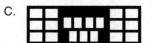 8 anterior periapical radiographs with size #1 film
8 posterior periapical radiographs with size #2 film
4 bitewing radiographs (horizontal or vertical) with size #2 film

C. 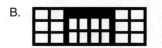 7 anterior periapical radiographs with size #1 film
8 posterior periapical radiographs with size #2 film
4 bitewing radiographs (horizontal or vertical) with size #2 film

D. 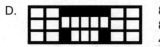 8 anterior periapical radiographs with size #1 film
8 posterior periapical radiographs with size #2 film
4 bitewing radiographs (horizontal or vertical) with size #2 film

Figure 3.2 Four examples of full mouth series.

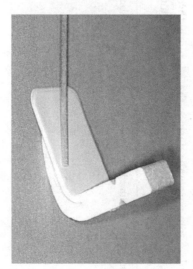

Figure 3.3 Place the embossed identification dot into the film retention groove of the film holder when placing a periapical film packet intraorally to keep it away from the area of interest, which is the root apices.

4. Place and expose the anterior periapical radiographs in the following order:

Full Mouth Series A

1st	right maxillary canine
2nd	maxillary central incisors
3rd	left maxillary canine
4th	left mandibular canine
5th	mandibular central incisors
6th	right mandibular canine

Full Mouth Series B

1st	right maxillary canine
2nd	right maxillary central-lateral incisors
3rd	left maxillary central-lateral incisors

4th	left maxillary canine
5th	left mandibular canine
6th	left mandibular central-lateral incisors
7th	right mandibular central-lateral incisors
8th	right mandibular canine

Note: Left-handed radiographers may use this order:

Full Mouth Series A

1st	left maxillary canine
2nd	maxillary central incisors
3rd	right maxillary canine
4th	right mandibular canine
5th	mandibular central incisors
6th	left mandibular canine

Full Mouth Series B

1st	left maxillary canine
2nd	left maxillary central-lateral incisors
3rd	right maxillary central-lateral incisors
4th	right maxillary canine
5th	right mandibular canine
6th	right mandibular central-lateral incisors
7th	left mandibular central-lateral incisors
8th	left mandibular canine

5. Process the films.

Part 2: Periapical Radiographs Using the Paralleling Technique—Posterior Region

1. Obtain eight size #2 film packets. All full mouth series configurations on adult patients will most likely use the same standard eight posterior film placements.

2. Place film into the Stabe® film holder with the long dimension positioned horizontally. (Figure 3.1)

3. Check posted exposure settings for the dental x-ray unit prior to placing each film packet, and set for the posterior region; adjust as needed for the maxilla and the mandible and for the premolar and molar regions.

4. Place and expose the posterior periapical radiographs in the following order:

1st	right maxillary premolar
2nd	right maxillary molar
3rd	right mandibular premolar
4th	right mandibular molar

5th	left maxillary premolar
6th	left maxillary molar
7th	left mandibular premolar
8th	left mandibular molar

Note: Left-handed radiographers may use this order:

1st	left maxillary premolar
2nd	left maxillary molar
3rd	left mandibular premolar
4th	left mandibular molar
5th	right maxillary premolar
6th	right maxillary molar
7th	right mandibular premolar
8th	right mandibular molar

5. Process the films.

COMPETENCY AND EVALUATION

1. Mount the processed films on the simulated film mount at the end of this chapter. Secure with a piece of tape placed along the top edge of the film only, so that the films may be raised slightly, to allow light underneath for ease of viewing. The use of removable transparent tape will allow the film mount page to be used more than once.

    NOTE: Use the labial mounting method. (See Laboratory Exercise 8, Film Mounting and Radiographic Landmarks, for details.) The raised portion of the embossed dot is toward you (convex) when placing the film onto the page.

2. Place the page with the mounted films taped to it on a view box and evaluate for acceptability. Circle the ✓ where packet placement, vertical angulation, horizontal angulation, and centering were performed correctly, and the ✗ where performed incorrectly. Identify which error was made by placing an ✗ on the corresponding line.

3. Obtain instructor feedback. Identify which step (packet placement, vertical angulation, horizontal angulation, centering) needs improvement.

4. Repeat Part 1 and Part 2 at the direction of your instructor. The film mount page may be copied to accommodate multiple practice attempts to achieve competency.

5. Having practiced the four steps of packet placement, vertical and horizontal angulation, and centering the x-ray beam, looking back over your self-evaluations, are there any consistencies? Which step do you feel most comfortable with? Which step do you feel needs improvement? What steps can you take to improve? Save these radiographs obtained utilizing the paralleling technique for comparison with the radiographs you expose using the bisecting technique in Laboratory Exercise 4, Periapical Radiographs—Bisecting Technique.

6. Complete the study questions.

Full Mouth Series A
Part 1: Anterior Periapical Radiographs—Maxilla
Mount Films Below

patient's right   patient's left

Right maxillary canine

packet placement   ✓ ✗
___ too far anterior
___ too far posterior

vertical angulation   ✓ ✗
___ excessive
___ inadequate

horizontal angulation ✓ ✗
___ from the mesial
___ from the distal

centering the PID   ✓ ✗
___ too far anterior
___ too far posterior
___ too far superior
___ too far inferior

Maxillary central incisors

packet placement   ✓ ✗
___ too far anterior
___ too far posterior

vertical angulation   ✓ ✗
___ excessive
___ inadequate

horizontal angulation ✓ ✗
___ from the mesial
___ from the distal

centering the PID   ✓ ✗
___ too far anterior
___ too far posterior
___ too far superior
___ too far inferior

Left maxillary canine

packet placement   ✓ ✗
___ too far anterior
___ too far posterior

vertical angulation   ✓ ✗
___ excessive
___ inadequate

horizontal angulation ✓ ✗
___ from the mesial
___ from the distal

centering the PID   ✓ ✗
___ too far anterior
___ too far posterior
___ too far superior
___ too far inferior

NAME _____

Full Mouth Series A

Part 1: Anterior Periapical Radiographs—Mandible

Mount Films Below

patient's right   patient's left

Right mandibular canine

packet placement   ✓ ✗
___ too far anterior
___ too far posterior

vertical angulation   ✓ ✗
___ excessive
___ inadequate

horizontal angulation ✓ ✗
___ from the mesial
___ from the distal

centering the PID   ✓ ✗
___ too far anterior
___ too far posterior
___ too far superior
___ too far inferior

Mandibular central-incisors

packet placement   ✓ ✗
___ too far anterior
___ too far posterior

vertical angulation   ✓ ✗
___ excessive
___ inadequate

horizontal angulation ✓ ✗
___ from the mesial
___ from the distal

centering the PID   ✓ ✗
___ too far anterior
___ too far posterior
___ too far superior
___ too far inferior

Left mandibular canine

packet placement   ✓ ✗
___ too far anterior
___ too far posterior

vertical angulation   ✓ ✗
___ excessive
___ inadequate

horizontal angulation ✓ ✗
___ from the mesial
___ from the distal

centering the PID   ✓ ✗
___ too far anterior
___ too far posterior
___ too far superior
___ too far inferior

NAME _____

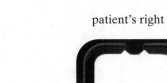

Full Mouth Series B
Part 1: Anterior Periapical Radiographs—Maxilla
Mount Films Below

patient's right   patient's left

Right maxillary canine	**Right maxillary central-lateral incisors**	**Left maxillary central-lateral incisors**	**Left maxillary canine**
packet placement ✓ ✗	**packet placement** ✓ ✗	**packet placement** ✓ ✗	**packet placement** ✓ ✗
___ too far anterior	___ too far anterior	___ too far anterior	___ too far anterior
___ too far posterior	___ too far posterior	___ too far posterior	___ too far posterior
vertical angulation ✓ ✗	**vertical angulation** ✓ ✗	**vertical angulation** ✓ ✗	**vertical angulation** ✓ ✗
___ excessive	___ excessive	___ excessive	___ excessive
___ inadequate	___ inadequate	___ inadequate	___ inadequate
horizontal angulation ✓ ✗	**horizontal angulation** ✓ ✗	**horizontal angulation** ✓ ✗	**horizontal angulation** ✓ ✗
___ from the mesial	___ from the mesial	___ from the mesial	___ from the mesial
___ from the distal	___ from the distal	___ from the distal	___ from the distal
centering the PID ✓ ✗	**centering the PID** ✓ ✗	**centering the PID** ✓ ✗	**centering the PID** ✓ ✗
___ too far anterior	___ too far anterior	___ too far anterior	___ too far anterior
___ too far posterior	___ too far posterior	___ too far posterior	___ too far posterior
___ too far superior	___ too far superior	___ too far superior	___ too far superior
___ too far inferior	___ too far inferior	___ too far inferior	___ too far inferior

Full Mouth Series B
Part 1: Anterior Periapical Radiographs—Mandible
Mount Films Below

patient's right   patient's left

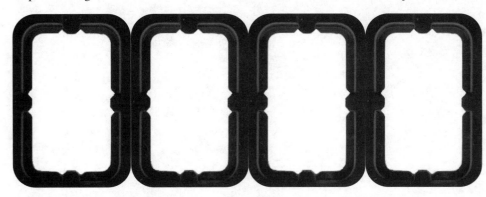

Right mandibular canine	**Right mandibular central-lateral incisors**	**Left mandibular central-lateral incisors**	**Left mandibular canine**
packet placement ✓ ✗	**packet placement** ✓ ✗	**packet placement** ✓ ✗	**packet placement** ✓ ✗
___ too far anterior	___ too far anterior	___ too far anterior	___ too far anterior
___ too far posterior	___ too far posterior	___ too far posterior	___ too far posterior
vertical angulation ✓ ✗	**vertical angulation** ✓ ✗	**vertical angulation** ✓ ✗	**vertical angulation** ✓ ✗
___ excessive	___ excessive	___ excessive	___ excessive
___ inadequate	___ inadequate	___ inadequate	___ inadequate
horizontal angulation ✓ ✗	**horizontal angulation** ✓ ✗	**horizontal angulation** ✓ ✗	**horizontal angulation** ✓ ✗
___ from the mesial	___ from the mesial	___ from the mesial	___ from the mesial
___ from the distal	___ from the distal	___ from the distal	___ from the distal
centering the PID ✓ ✗	**centering the PID** ✓ ✗	**centering the PID** ✓ ✗	**centering the PID** ✓ ✗
___ too far anterior	___ too far anterior	___ too far anterior	___ too far anterior
___ too far posterior	___ too far posterior	___ too far posterior	___ too far posterior
___ too far superior	___ too far superior	___ too far superior	___ too far superior
___ too far inferior	___ too far inferior	___ too far inferior	___ too far inferior

Full Mouth Series A and B
Part 2: Posterior Periapical Radiographs
Mount Films Below

patient's right side

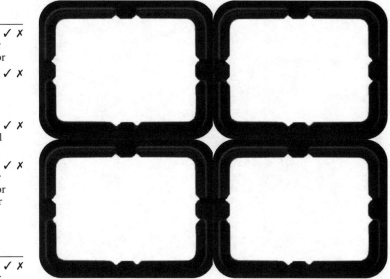

Right maxillary molar

packet placement ✓ ✗
___ too far anterior
___ too far posterior

vertical angulation ✓ ✗
___ excessive
___ inadequate

horizontal angulation ✓ ✗
___ from the mesial
___ from the distal

centering the PID ✓ ✗
___ too far anterior
___ too far posterior
___ too far superior
___ too far inferior

Right maxillary premolar

packet placement ✓ ✗
___ too far anterior
___ too far posterior

vertical angulation ✓ ✗
___ excessive
___ inadequate

horizontal angulation ✓ ✗
___ from the mesial
___ from the distal

centering the PID ✓ ✗
___ too far anterior
___ too far posterior
___ too far superior
___ too far inferior

Right mandibular molar

packet placement ✓ ✗
___ too far anterior
___ too far posterior

vertical angulation ✓ ✗
___ excessive
___ inadequate

horizontal angulation ✓ ✗
___ from the mesial
___ from the distal

centering the PID ✓ ✗
___ too far anterior
___ too far posterior
___ too far superior
___ too far inferior

Right mandibular premolar

packet placement ✓ ✗
___ too far anterior
___ too far posterior

vertical angulation ✓ ✗
___ excessive
___ inadequate

horizontal angulation ✓ ✗
___ from the mesial
___ from the distal

centering the PID ✓ ✗
___ too far anterior
___ too far posterior
___ too far superior
___ too far inferior

Full Mouth Series A and B
Part 2: Posterior Periapical Radiographs
Mount Films Below

patient's left side

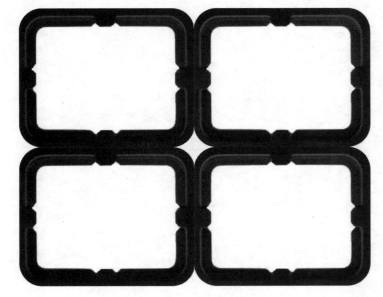

Left maxillary premolar

packet placement ✓ ✗
___ too far anterior
___ too far posterior

vertical angulation ✓ ✗
___ excessive
___ inadequate

horizontal angulation ✓ ✗
___ from the mesial
___ from the distal

centering the PID ✓ ✗
___ too far anterior
___ too far posterior
___ too far superior
___ too far inferior

Left maxillary molar

packet placement ✓ ✗
___ too far anterior
___ too far posterior

vertical angulation ✓ ✗
___ excessive
___ inadequate

horizontal angulation ✓ ✗
___ from the mesial
___ from the distal

centering the PID ✓ ✗
___ too far anterior
___ too far posterior
___ too far superior
___ too far inferior

Left mandibular premolar

packet placement ✓ ✗
___ too far anterior
___ too far posterior

vertical angulation ✓ ✗
___ excessive
___ inadequate

horizontal angulation ✓ ✗
___ from the mesial
___ from the distal

centering the PID ✓ ✗
___ too far anterior
___ too far posterior
___ too far superior
___ too far inferior

Left mandibular molar

packet placement ✓ ✗
___ too far anterior
___ too far posterior

vertical angulation ✓ ✗
___ excessive
___ inadequate

horizontal angulation ✓ ✗
___ from the mesial
___ from the distal

centering the PID ✓ ✗
___ too far anterior
___ too far posterior
___ too far superior
___ too far inferior

I. Periapical radiographs
  A. Uses
    1. Suspected periapical condition
    2. Trauma or injury to the teeth
    3. Periodontal involvement
    4. Endodontic therapy
    5. Large carious lesions
    6. Suspected impactions
    7. Unusual eruption pattern, malpositioned or unexplained missing teeth
    8. Unexplained pain
    9. Unusual tooth morphology/color
    10. Evaluation of implants
  B. Types
    1. Anterior
      a. Intraoral film packet size #1 or size #2 or a combination of both are typically used when exposing anterior periapical radiographs on adults and adolescents after the eruption of the second permanent molars. Anterior periapical radiographs on children with primary dentition (3 to 6 years of age) use intraoral film packet size #0; and children with transitional (mixed primary and permanent) dentition use size #0 or size #1.
      b. The number and location of placement of film packets varies among practices.
      c. The long dimension of the film packet is placed vertically in the oral cavity.
    2. Posterior
      a. Intraoral film packet size #2 is typically used when exposing posterior periapical radiographs on adults and adolescents after the eruption of the second permanent molars. Posterior periapical radiographs on children with primary dentition (3 to 6 years of age) use intraoral film packet size #0 or size #1; and children with transitional (mixed primary and permanent) dentition use size #1 or size #2.
      b. The number and location of placement of film packets is the same among practices.
      c. The long dimension of the film packet is placed horizontally in the mouth.
II. Paralleling technique
  A. Principle concepts
    1. White unprinted side of the film packet is placed toward the teeth.
    2. The embossed identification dot is positioned away from the area of interest. (Place "dot in the slot" of the film holder to position toward the incisal/occlusal edge and away from the apices of the teeth.)
    3. Film is placed parallel to the teeth being imaged. To achieve parallelism, film must be placed well into the oral cavity, toward

the midsaggittal plane, increasing the distance between the film and tooth.

    a. The film holder used with the paralleling technique must have a long bite block to allow for parallel placement of the film packet.

    b. When utilizing the Stabe® film-holding device, the teeth must occlude on the bite block extension to achieve a parallel relationship between the long axes of the teeth and the plane of the film packet. EXCEPTION: In the mandibular posterior region, the bite extension may be removed to shorten the holder for ease of placement in the oral cavity. (Figure 3.4 ■)

4. A long PID (12″ or 16″) should be used to minimize distortion which results when the film-to-tooth distance is increased.

5. Central ray of the x-ray beam is directed perpendicular, toward the center of the film.

6. Film is held in place by a bite block or other periapical film-holding device.

  B. Advantages

    1. Provides quality images with minimal geometric distortion

    2. Minimizes the superimposition of adjacent structures

    3. Potential standardization of subsequent radiographs

  C. Disadvantages

    1. Packet placement may be uncomfortable for the patient to tolerate.

    2. True parallel placement may be difficult for the radiographer to achieve.

    3. A long 12″ or 16″ PID should be used for best results.

III. Periapical radiographic procedure—anterior region

  A. Placement of the film packet (*Full Mouth Series A*) (Figure 3.5 ■)

    1. Maxillary central incisors periapical radiograph

      a. Align the film packet so that the maxillary central and lateral incisors on both the right and left sides are centered in the middle of the film packet.

      b. Ensure that the film packet is placed such that the entire maxillary central and lateral incisors and the mesial half of both the right and left canines will be recorded on the film.

      c. Place the film packet parallel to the central and lateral incisors.

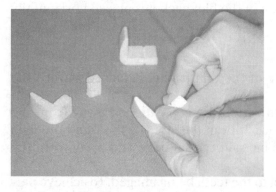

Figure 3.4 The Stabe® holder bite extension may be removed to shorten the holder when utilizing the bisecting technique. When using the paralleling technique, a shortened Stabe® film holder may also be used in the mandibular posterior regions *only*.

Maxillary Central-Lateral Incisors   Maxillary Canine

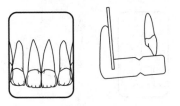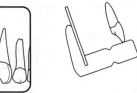

Mandibular Central-Lateral Incisors   Mandibular Canine

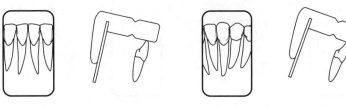

Figure 3.5 Full mouth series A—Film packet placement for anterior periapical radiographs.

2. Maxillary canine periapical radiograph
   a. Align the film packet so that the maxillary canine is centered in the middle of the film packet.
   b. Ensure that the film packet is placed such that the maxillary distal half of the lateral, entire canine, and the mesial half of the first premolar will be recorded on the film.
   c. Place the film packet parallel to the canine.
3. Mandibular central incisors periapical radiograph
   a. Align the film packet so that the mandibular central and lateral incisors on both the right and left sides are centered in the middle of the film packet.
   b. Ensure that the film packet is placed such that the entire mandibular central incisors and lateral incisors and the mesial half of both the right and left canines will be recorded on the film.
   c. Place the film packet parallel to the central and lateral incisors.
4. Mandibular canine periapical radiograph
   a. Align the film packet so that the mandibular canine is centered in the middle of the film packet.
   b. Ensure that the film packet is placed such that the mandibular distal half of the lateral, entire canine, and the mesial half of the first premolar will be recorded on the film.
   c. Place the film packet parallel to the canine.
B. Placement of the film packet—*Full Mouth Series B* (Figure 3.6 ■)
   1. Maxillary central-lateral incisors periapical radiograph
      a. Align the film packet so that the maxillary central and lateral incisors on one side are centered in the middle of the film packet.
      b. Ensure that the film packet is placed such that the maxillary distal half of the central incisor on the opposite side, the entire central and lateral incisors on the side being imaged, and the mesial half of the canine will be recorded on the film.
      c. Place the film packet parallel to the central and lateral incisors.

Maxillary Central-Lateral Incisors   Maxillary Canine

  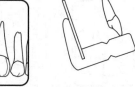

Mandibular Central-Lateral Incisors   Mandibular Canine

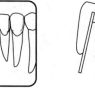 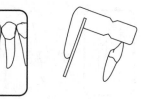

Figure 3.6 Full mouth series B—Film packet placement for anterior periapical radiographs.

2. Maxillary canine periapical radiograph
   a. Align the film packet so that the maxillary canine is centered in the middle of the film packet.
   b. Ensure that the film packet is placed such that the maxillary distal half of the lateral, entire canine, and the mesial half of the first premolar will be recorded on the film.
   c. Place the film packet parallel to the canine.

3. Mandibular central-lateral incisors periapical radiograph
   a. Align the film packet so that the mandibular lateral and central incisors on one side are centered in the middle of the film packet.
   b. Ensure that the film packet is placed such that the mandibular distal half of the central incisor on the opposite side, the entire central and lateral incisors on the side being imaged, and the mesial half of the canine will be recorded on the film.
   c. Place the film packet parallel to the central and lateral incisors.

4. Mandibular canine periapical radiograph
   a. Align the film packet so that the mandibular canine is centered in the middle of the film packet.
   b. Ensure that the film packet is placed such that the mandibular distal half of the lateral, entire canine, and the mesial half of the first premolar will be recorded on the film.
   c. Place the film packet parallel to the canine.

IV. Periapical radiographic procedure—Posterior region
   A. Placement of the film packet—*Same for all full mouth series configurations* (Figure 3.7 ■)
      1. Maxillary premolar periapical radiograph
         a. Align the mesial edge of the film packet far enough forward to line up behind the middle of the maxillary canine.
         b. Ensure that the film packet is placed such that the maxillary distal half of the canine, first and second premolars, first molar, and mesial half of the second molar will be recorded on the film.
         c. Place the film packet parallel to the premolars.

Figure 3.7 Film packet placement for posterior periapical radiographs. When placing the film packet in the posterior region of the mandible, the Stabe® film holder bite extension may be removed. A Stabe® holder shortened in this way will fit more comfortably in this area. *Do not* remove the bite extension in any other region when using this holder with the paralleling technique. The extension is necessary for parallel relationship between tooth and plane of the film in all other areas.

Maxillary Premolar   Maxillary Molar

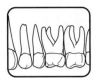 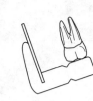

Mandibular Premolar   Mandibular Molar

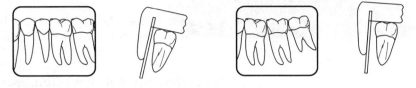

2. Maxillary molar periapical radiograph
   a. Align the mesial edge of the film packet behind the middle of the maxillary second premolar.
   b. Ensure that the film packet is placed such that the maxillary distal half of the second premolar and the first, second, and third molar will be recorded on the film.
   c. Place the film packet parallel to the molars.
3. Mandibular premolar periapical radiograph
   a. Align the mesial edge of the film packet far enough forward to line up behind the middle of the mandibular canine.
   b. Ensure that the film packet is placed such that the mandibular distal half of the canine, first and second premolars, first molar, and mesial half of the second molar will be recorded on the film.
   c. Place the film packet parallel to the premolars.
4. Mandibular molar periapical radiograph
   a. Align the mesial edge of the film packet behind the middle of the mandibular second premolar.
   b. Ensure that the film packet is placed such that the mandibular distal half of the second premolar and first, second, and third molar will be recorded on the film.
   c. Place the film packet parallel to the molars.
V. Vertical Angulation
   A. Determine the up and down angulation of the PID. Positive angulation is achieved by pointing the PID down toward the floor. Generally, maxillary periapical radiographs will require a positive vertical angulation, and mandibular periapical radiographs will usually require a negative vertical angulation.
   B. Direct the x-ray beam to intersect the film perpendicularly in the vertical dimension. (Figure 3.8 ■) As a visual aid in determining

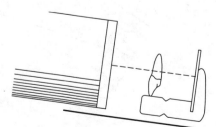

Figure 3.8 Vertical angulation for periapical radiographs should be such that the beam will intersect the film perpendicularly in the vertical dimension. Note the line drawn to indicate that the vertical slant of the PID is parallel to the vertical slant of the extension of the film holder.

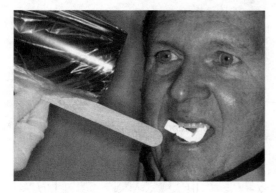

Figure 3.9 Use of a tongue blade acts as a visual aid in determining the correct vertical angulation.

the correct vertical angulation, use a tongue blade as an extension of the Stabe® bite block film holder; align the vertical angle of the PID parallel to the tongue blade in the vertical dimension. (Figure 3.9 ■)

VI. Horizontal Angulation
   A. Horizontal angulation of the x-ray beam
      1. Determine the side-to-side placement of the PID.
      2. Align the PID such that the central ray of the x-ray beam will intersect the film perpendicularly. Perpendicular alignment of the beam can be achieved either of two ways:
         a. Direct the central ray of the x-ray beam through a predetermined interproximal space or directly at the tooth being imaged. Examine the contact points of the patient's teeth to determine the correct horizontal angulation. Use the following guidelines (Figure 3.10 ■):
            1) For the central incisors periapical radiograph, direct the central ray of the x-ray beam between the right and left central incisors.
            2) For the central-lateral incisors periapical radiograph, direct the central ray of the x-ray beam between the central incisor and lateral incisor.

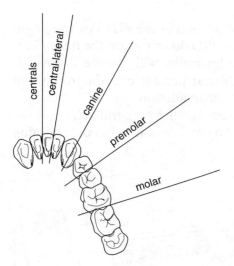

Figure 3.10 Horizontal angulation for central incisors, central-lateral incisors, canine, premolar, and molar periapical radiographs can be determined by directing the central ray of the x-ray beam between a predetermined interproximal space.

3) For the canine periapical radiograph, direct the central ray of the x-ray beam directly at the middle of the canine.

4) For the premolar periapical radiograph, direct the central ray between the first and second premolars.

5) For the molar periapical radiograph, direct the central ray between the first and second molars.

b. Using the open end of the PID as the reference point, align such that the open end of the PID is parallel to the film in the horizontal plane. Visualizing the horizontal placement of the PID is easily achieved by placing a tongue blade across the open end and rotating the tube head horizontally until the tongue blade and, hence, the open end of the PID, is parallel to the film. (Figure 3.11 ■)

VII. Centering the x-ray beam over the film packet

A. Determine the placement of the film packet. Use any part of the film holder that is visible outside the mouth as an indication of where the film packet is located.

B. Direct the central rays of the x-ray beam toward the center of the film.

C. Using the Stabe® film holder as a reference point, align the PID directly over the film packet. The film will usually be centered in the diameter of the PID when the edge of the PID is positioned 1/4″ beyond the holder edge. (Figure 3.12 ■) Correct placement of the PID can be achieved by placing the tongue blade as an extension of the PID. No part of the film packet should be visible beyond the diameter of the PID when extending the tongue blade. (Figure 3.13 ■)

VIII. Errors

A. Packet placement error

1. Occurs when the film packet is not placed correctly intraorally

2. Results in the appropriate teeth not being imaged on the film

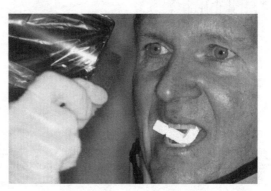

Figure 3.11 Use of a tongue blade acts as a visual aid in determining the correct horizontal angulation.

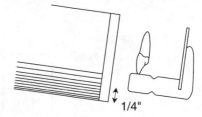

1/4"

Figure 3.12 The PID will be centered over the film packet when the edge of the PID is aligned into position 1/4″ below the Stabe® film holder bite extension.

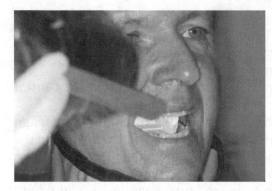

Figure 3.13 Use of tongue blade acts as a visual aid in determining centering of the x-ray beam over the film packet.

          3. Packet placed too far anteriorly (Figure 3.14 ■)
          4. Packet placed too far posteriorly (Figure 3.15 ■)
     B. Vertical angulation error
          1. Occurs when the up-and-down angle of the PID is not set such that the x-ray beam intersects the film perpendicularly in the vertical plane
          2. Results in the incisal/occlusal edges or the apcies of the teeth not being imaged on the film
            NOTE: If an elongation or foreshortening error is noted (see Laboratory Exercise 4, Periapical Radiographs—Bisecting Technique), then the film was not placed in the mouth correctly. When placing the film packet parallel to the teeth, it is geometrically impossible to get elongation or foreshortening error.
          3. Excessive vertical angulation when utilizing the paralleling technique results in the incisal/occlusal edge being cut off the resultant image (Figure 3.16 ■)

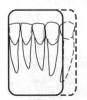

Figure 3.14 A mandibular central-lateral incisors periapical radiograph with film packet placed too far anteriorly so as not to image the contact between the lateral incisor and the canine.

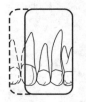

Figure 3.15 A maxillary central-lateral incisors periapical radiograph with film packet placed too far posteriorly so as not to image the contact between the right and left central incisors.

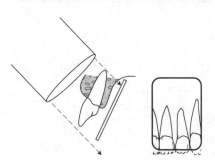

Figure 3.16 When utilizing the paralleling technique, excessive vertical angulation results in incisal/occlusal edges being cut off the image.

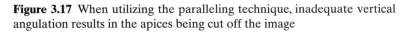

Figure 3.17 When utilizing the paralleling technique, inadequate vertical angulation results in the apices being cut off the image

      4. Inadequate vertical angulation when utilizing the paralleling technique results in the apices edge being cut off the resultant image (Figure 3.17 ■)

C. Horizontal angulation error

      1. Occurs when the side-to-side angulation of the PID is not set such that the beam will intersect with the film perpendicularly

      2. Results in superimposition of proximal surfaces of adjacent teeth (overlap error)

      3. Occurs when the beam intersects with the film obliquely from the mesial direction (Figure 3.18 ■)

      4. Occurs when the beam intersects with the film obliquely from the distal direction (Figure 3.19 ■)

D. Centering the x-ray beam over the film error

      1. Occurs when the PID is not placed directly over the film packet

      2. Results in an unexposed or clear area (cone-cut error) recorded on the film

      3. Creates a cone-cut error when the beam is too far toward the anterior (Figure 3.20 ■)

      4. Creates a cone-cut error when the beam is too far toward the posterior (Figure 3.21 ■)

      5. Creates a cone-cut error when the beam is too far toward the superior (Figure 3.22 ■)

      6. Creates a cone-cut error when the beam is too far toward the inferior (Figure 3.23 ■)

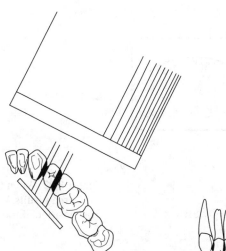

Figure 3.18 When horizontal angulation intersects the film packet obliquely from the mesial, the most severe overlap occurs in the posterior region of the image.

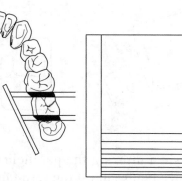

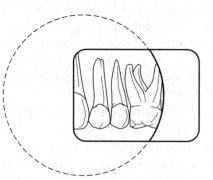

Figure 3.19 When horizontal angulation intersects the film packet obliquely from the distal, the most severe overlap occurs in the anterior region of the image.

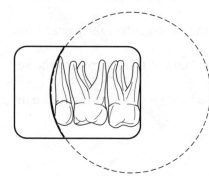

Figure 3.20 When the PID is not centered over the film, an unexposed or clear "cone-cut" area results. When the cone-cut is in the posterior section of the image, the PID was positioned too far anterior.

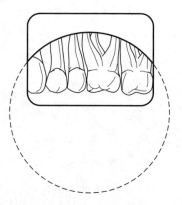

Figure 3.21 When the PID is not centered over the film, an unexposed or clear "cone-cut" area results. When the cone-cut is in the anterior section of the image, the PID was positioned too far posterior.

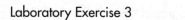

Figure 3.22 When the PID is not centered over the film, an unexposed or clear "cone-cut" area results. When the cone-cut is in the inferior section of the image, the PID was positioned too far superior.

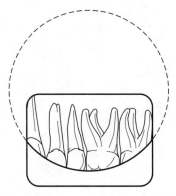

Figure 3.23 When the PID is not centered over the film, an unexposed or clear "cone-cut" area results. When the cone-cut is in the superior section of the image, the PID was positioned too far inferior.

BIBLIOGRAPHY

ADA Council on Scientific Affairs. An update on radiographic practices: Information and recommendations. *Journal of the American Dental Association* 2001;132:234–238.

Haring, JI, Howerton, LJ. *Dental Radiography. Principles and Techniques,* 3rd ed. St. Louis, MO: Elsevier; 2006: 181–212.

Johnson, ON, Thomson, EM. *Essentials of Dental Radiography for Dental Assistants and Hygienists,* 8th ed. Upper Saddle River, NJ: Prentice Hall; 2007: 137–179.

Miles, DA, VanDis, ML, Jensen, CW, Ferretti, AB. *Radiographic Imaging for the Dental Auxiliaries,* 3rd ed. St. Louis, MO: Elsevier; 1999: 9–40.

Thomson, EM. Dental radiographs for the child client. *Dental Hygienist News;* 1993; 6:19–20, 24.

1. How many posterior periapical radiographs are exposed in a standard adult full mouth series?
    - A. 4
    - B. 6
    - C. 8
    - D. 10

2. Which of the following teeth should be imaged on a mandibular canine periapical radiograph?
    - A. Distal portion of the central incisor, lateral incisor, mesial portion of the canine
    - B. Distal portion of the lateral incisor, canine, mesial portion of the first premolar
    - C. Distal portion of the canine, first premolar, mesial portion of the second premolar
    - D. Distal portion of the first premolar, second premolar, mesial portion of the first molar

3. Which of the following teeth should be imaged on a maxillary premolar periapical radiograph?
    - A. Distal portion of the central incisor, lateral incisor, canine, first premolar, mesial portion of the second premolar
    - B. Distal portion of the lateral incisor, canine, first premolar, second premolar, mesial portion of the first molar
    - C. Distal portion of the canine, first premolar, second premolar, first molar, mesial portion of the second molar
    - D. Distal portion of the second premolar, first molar, second molar, third molar

4. To avoid horizontal overlap error, through which interproximal space should the central ray of the x-ray beam be directed when exposing a mandibular *molar* periapical radiograph?
    - A. Between the canine and the first premolar
    - B. Between the first premolar and the second premolar
    - C. Between the second premolar and the first molar
    - D. Between the first molar and the second molar
    - E. Between the second molar and the third molar

5. To avoid horizontal overlap error, through which interproximal space should the central ray of the x-ray beam be directed when exposing a maxillary *premolar* periapical radiograph?
    - A. Between the canine and the first premolar
    - B. Between the first premolar and the second premolar
    - C. Between the second premolar and the first molar
    - D. Between the first molar and the second molar
    - E. Between the second molar and the third molar

6. A mandibular molar periapical radiograph that did not image the entire third molar results from an error made in which of the following?
    A. Packet placement
    B. Vertical angulation
    C. Horizontal angulation
    D. Centering the x-ray beam

7. Referring to question 6, which of the following would correct this error?
    A. Position the film packet more posteriorly
    B. Increase vertical angulation
    C. Shift the horizontal angulation toward the mesial
    D. Direct the PID more toward the posterior

8. Not imaging the apices of the teeth results from an error made in which of the following?
    A. Packet placement
    B. Vertical angulation
    C. Horizontal angulation
    D. Centering the x-ray beam

9. Referring to question 8, which of the following would correct this error?
    A. Position the film packet more superiorly
    B. Increase vertical angulation
    C. Shift the horizontal angulation toward the distal
    D. Direct the PID more toward the anterior

10. A premolar periapical radiograph which is undiagnostic due to overlapped interproximal areas is the result of incorrect:
    A. Packet placement
    B. Vertical angulation
    C. Horizontal angulation
    D. Centering of the x-ray beam

Periapical Radiographs— Bisecting Technique

INTRODUCTION

The American Dental Association and the American Academy of Oral and Maxillofacial Radiology recommend using the paralleling technique when exposing intraoral radiographs. However, it is not always possible to achieve the ideal parallel film packet placement on every patient. Parallelism is difficult to achieve in patients who present with a shallow palatal vault, such as found in children, or when large palatal or mandibular tori are present. When the paralleling technique is not feasible, quality radiographic images may still be acquired if the radiographer has mastered the bisecting technique.

Use of the bisecting technique does not alter the size and number of films required for a full mouth series of radiographs. Additionally, the same four steps of packet placement, vertical angulation, horizontal angulation, and centering the x-ray beam are followed when utilizing either technique. The major differences between the paralleling and bisecting techniques are (1) the film packet position in relationship to the teeth and (2) the vertical angulation of the PID required to compensate for this position. When using the paralleling technique, the film packet is placed parallel to the long axis of the tooth, whereas, when employing the bisecting technique, the film packet is placed as close to the tooth as possible without regard to a parallel relationship. The film packet may even contact the lingual surface of the tooth. Because the film and tooth are not parallel, the central rays of the x-ray beam cannot be directed to perpendicularly intersect both the film and the long axis of the tooth. Instead, when using the bisecting technique, the vertical angulation must be directed perpendicular to the imaginary bisector—a plane between the film plane and the long axis of the tooth. A general rule of thumb is that an increased vertical angulation is required in the bisecting technique over that used for the paralleling technique. (Figure 4.1 ■)

There are a variety of commercially made film-holding devices on the market for use with the bisecting technique. This exercise uses the Stabe® (Dentsply Rinn) (Figure 4.2 ■) disposable, polystyrene bite block film holder, but the student may be directed to complete the activity using the

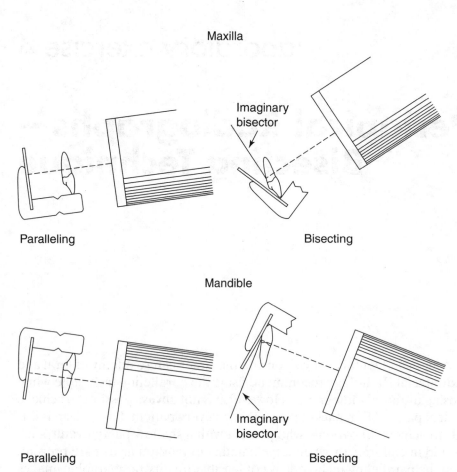

Maxilla

Imaginary bisector

Paralleling   Bisecting

Mandible

Imaginary bisector

Paralleling   Bisecting

Figure 4.1 A comparison of the vertical angulation used when utilizing the paralleling and bisecting techniques.

standard film-holding device at his/her institution. The Stabe® film holder (used in Laboratory Exercise 3, Periapical Radiographs—Paralleling Technique) has the advantage of being adaptable, with a slight modification to be used with both the paralleling and the bisecting techniques. A thorough understanding of film packet placement and vertical and horizontal beam angulation is needed to master the bisecting technique. The Stabe® periapical film holder allows the student to develop the skills and ability to determine appropriate angles without relying on an external aiming device. By creating this need to know correct angles and accurate image geometry, the student gains basic skills that may be carried over to any type of film

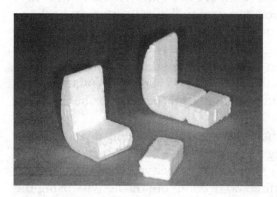

Figure 4.2 Stabe® film holder modified for use with the bisecting technique.

holder. (See Laboratory Exercise 5, Radiographic Techniques with Supplemental Film Holders.)

OBJECTIVES

Following the completion of this lab activity, you will be able to:

1. Alter the Stabe® film-holding device for use with the bisecting technique.

2. Demonstrate proficiency in placing, exposing, and processing anterior and posterior periapical radiographs using the bisecting technique.

3. Critique a full mouth series consisting of anterior and posterior periapicals for correct (a) placement of the film packet intraorally; (b) vertical and (c) horizontal angulation of the PID; and (d) exposure of the film by directing the x-ray beam over the film packet.

MATERIALS

Teaching manikin or skull

Lead (or lead equivalent) apron and thyroid collar

Size #1 and size #2 radiographic films

Periapical film-holding device (disposable Stabe® film holders or similar device designed for use with the bisecting technique)

Viewbox

Tongue blades

PREPARATION

1. Study the chapter outline to prepare for this laboratory exercise. An understanding of the material presented in the outline is required to complete this activity.

2. Utilize Table 4.1 to assist you with completing the exercises. Instructor demonstration may enhance knowledge of the laboratory exercise.

3. Prepare radiology operatory. Set up teaching manikin or skull. Ensure that correct "patient" positioning is achieved. To image the maxilla, ensure that the maxillary occlusal plane is parallel to the floor; to image the mandible, ensure that the mandibular occlusal plane is parallel to the floor and the mid-sagittal plane must be perpendicular to the floor for both maxillary and mandibular exposures.

4. Place lead apron (or lead-equivalent barrier) and thyroid collar over the "patient."

5. The size and/or number of films included in a full mouth series of periapical radiographs varies among practices. The anterior periapical radiographic examination may include the exposure of 6, 7, or 8 periapical radiographs, whereas the posterior radiographic examination

TABLE 4.1 Film Packet Placement, Vertical and Horizontal Angulation, and Centering for Anterior and Posterior Periapical Radiographs for Adult Patients Utilizing the Bisecting Technique

Periapical Radiograph	Film Packet Placement	Vertical Angulation*	Horizontal Angulation	Centering*
Maxillary Central Incisors Use film size #1 or size #2	Center the film packet to line up behind the central and lateral incisors on both the right and left sides; if using a size #2 film, include the mesial halves of the canines.	Direct the central rays of the x-ray beam toward the imaginary bisector between the long axes of the teeth and the film in the vertical dimension; +40 degrees	Direct the central rays of the x-ray beam perpendicularly through the left and right central incisor embrasure.	Center the film packet within the x-ray beam; direct the central rays of the x-ray beam toward the center of the film at point near the tip of the nose.
Maxillary Central-Lateral Incisors Use film size #1	Center the film packet to line up behind the central and lateral incisors on one side of the mouth; include a portion of the central incisor on the opposite side and a portion of the canine.	Direct the central rays of the x-ray beam toward the imaginary bisector between the long axes of the teeth and the film in the vertical dimension; +40 degrees	Direct the central rays of the x-ray beam perpendicularly through the central incisor and lateral incisor embrasure.	Center the film packet within the x-ray beam; direct the central rays of the x-ray beam toward the center of the film at a point between the root tips of the central incisor and the canine.
Maxillary Canine Use film size #1 or size #2	Center the film packet to line up behind the canine; include the distal half of the lateral incisor and the mesial half of the first premolar.	Direct the central rays of the x-ray beam toward the imaginary bisector between the long axes of the teeth and the film in the vertical dimension; +45 degrees	Direct the central rays of the x-ray beam perpendicularly in the horizontal direction at the center of the canine.	Center the film packet within the x-ray beam; direct the central rays of the x-ray beam toward the center of the film at the root of the canine, near the ala (corner) of the nose.
Maxillary Premolar Use film size #2	Align the anterior edge of film packet to line up behind the distal half of the canine; include the first and second premolars, first molar, and mesial half of the second molar.	Direct the central rays of the x-ray beam toward the imaginary bisector between the long axes of the teeth and the film in the vertical dimension; +30 degrees	Direct the central rays of the x-ray beam perpendicularly through the first and second premolar embrasure.	Center the film packet within the x-ray beam; direct the central rays of the x-ray beam toward the center of the film at a point on the ala-tragus line (on the cheek bone) directly below the pupil of the eye.

	Packet Placement	Vertical Angulation	Horizontal Angulation	Point of Entry
Maxillary Molar Use film size #2	Align the anterior edge of film packet to line up behind the distal half of the second premolar; include the first, second, and third molars.	Direct the central rays of the x-ray beam toward the imaginary bisector between the long axes of the teeth and the film in the vertical dimension; +20 degrees	Direct the central rays of the x-ray beam perpendicularly through the first and second molar embrasure.	Center the film packet within the x-ray beam; direct the central rays of the x-ray beam toward the center of the film at a point on the ala-tragus line (on the cheek bone) directly below the outer canthus (corner) of the eye.
Mandibular Central Incisors Use film size #1 or size #2	Center the film packet to line up behind the central and lateral incisors; if using a size #2 film, include the mesial halves of the canines.	Direct the central rays of the x-ray beam toward the imaginary bisector between the long axes of the teeth and the film in the vertical dimension; −15 degrees.	Direct the central rays of the x-ray beam perpendicularly through the left and right central incisor embrasure.	Center the film packet within the x-ray beam; direct the central rays of the x-ray beam toward the center of the film at a point on the center of the chin 1 in. (2.5 cm) above the lower border of the mandible.
Mandibular Central-Lateral Incisors Use film size #1	Center the film packet to line up behind the central and lateral incisors on one side of the mouth; include a portion of the central incisor on the opposite side and a portion of the canine.	Direct the central rays of the x-ray beam toward the imaginary bisector between the long axes of the teeth and the film in the vertical dimension; −15 degrees.	Direct the central rays of the x-ray beam perpendicularly through the central incisor and lateral incisor embrasure.	Center the film packet within the x-ray beam; direct the central rays of the x-ray beam toward the center of the film at a point on the chin near the central and lateral root tips, 1 in. (2.5 cm) above the lower border of the mandible.
Mandibular Canine Use film size #1 or size #2	Center the film packet to line up behind the canine; include the distal half of the lateral incisor and the mesial half of the first premolar.	Direct the central rays of the x-ray beam toward the imaginary bisector between the long axes of the teeth and the film in the vertical dimension; −20 degrees	Direct the central rays of the x-ray beam perpendicularly in the horizontal direction at the center of the canine	Center the film packet within the x-ray beam; direct the central rays of the x-ray beam toward the center of the film at the center of the root of the canine; 1 in. (2.5 cm) above the inferior border of the mandible.

(continues)

TABLE 4.1 *(continued)*

Periapical Radiograph	Film Packet Placement	Vertical Angulation*	Horizontal Angulation	Centering*
Mandibular Premolar Use film size #2	Align the anterior edge of film packet to line up behind the distal half of the canine; include the first and second premolars, first molar, and mesial half of the second molar.	Direct the central rays toward the imaginary bisector between the long axes of the teeth and the film in the vertical dimension; −10 degrees.	Direct the central rays of the x-ray beam perpendicularly through the first and second premolar embrasure.	Center the film packet within the x-ray beam; direct the central rays of the x-ray beam toward the center of the film at a point on the chin 1 in. (2.5 cm) above the lower border of the mandible, directly inferior to the pupil of the eye.
Mandibular Molar Use film size #2	Align the anterior edge of film packet to line up behind the distal half of the second premolar; include the first, second, and third molars.	Direct the central rays of the x-ray beam toward the imaginary bisector between the long axes of the teeth and the film in the vertical dimension; −5 degrees.	Direct the central rays of the x-ray beam perpendicularly through the first and second molar embrasure	Center the film packet within the x-ray beam; direct the central rays of the x-ray beam toward the center of the film at a point on the chin 1 in. (2.5 cm) above the lower border of the mandible, directly below the outer canthus (corner) of the eye.

*The patient must be seated in the correct position with the occlusal plane of the arch being imaged parallel to the floor and the midsaggital plane perpendicular to the floor to use the vertical angulation and points of entry recommended by this chart.

Modified from *Essentials of Dental Radiography for Dental Assistants and Hygienists*, 8th ed. by O. N. Johnson and E. M. Thomson, Upper Saddle River, NJ: Prentice Hall, 2007: 167–168.

usually remains standard with the exposure of 8 periapical radiographs. (Figure 3.2) This exercise will focus on the use of two of the most common full mouth series configurations shown in Figures 3.2A and 3.2B in Laboratory Exercise 3, Periapical Radiographs—Paralleling Technique.

6. Obtain disposable Stabe® periapical film holders or similar device designed for use with the bisecting technique.

7. Orient the film packet in the film holder so that the embossed identification dot will be placed away from the apices of the teeth. Place the "dot in the slot" of the film holder to position the identification dot of the film packet toward the incisal/occlusal edges of the teeth.

8. Start with the anterior exposures. Beginning the examination with the more tolerable anterior film placements will help to gain the patient's confidence and cooperation with the procedure.

LABORATORY EXERCISE ACTIVITIES

Part 1: Periapical Radiographs Using the Bisecting Technique—Anterior Region

1. If using *Full Mouth Series A* for this exercise, you may choice to obtain six size #2 radiographic film packets or six size #1 radiographic film packets or a combination of five size #1 and one size #2 radiographic film packets. If using *Full Mouth Series B* for this exercise, obtain eight size #1 radiographic film packets.

2. Place film into the Stabe® film holder with the long dimension positioned vertically.

3. Check posted exposure factors for the dental x-ray unit prior to placing each film packet and set for the anterior region; adjust as needed for the maxilla and for the mandible and for the canine and the central incisor regions.

4. Place and expose the anterior periapical radiographs in the following order:

Full Mouth Series A

1st	right maxillary canine
2nd	maxillary central incisors
3rd	left maxillary canine
4th	left mandibular canine
5th	mandibular central incisors
6th	right mandibular canine

Full Mouth Series B

1st	right maxillary canine
2nd	right maxillary central-lateral incisors
3rd	left maxillary central-lateral incisors
4th	left maxillary canine

5th	left mandibular canine
6th	left mandibular central-lateral incisors
7th	right mandibular central-lateral incisors
8th	right mandibular canine

Note: Left-handed radiographers may use this order:

Full Mouth Series A

1st	left maxillary canine
2nd	maxillary central incisors
3rd	right maxillary canine
4th	right mandibular canine
5th	mandibular central incisors
6th	left mandibular canine

Full Mouth Series B

1st	left maxillary canine
2nd	left maxillary central-lateral incisors
3rd	right maxillary central-lateral incisors
4th	right maxillary canine
5th	right mandibular canine
6th	right mandibular central-lateral incisors
7th	left mandibular central-lateral incisors
8th	left mandibular canine

5. Process the films.

Part 2: Periapical Radiographs Using the Bisecting Technique—Posterior Region

1. Obtain eight size #2 film packets. All full mouth series configurations on adult patients will most likely use the same standard eight posterior film placements.

2. Place film into the Stabe® film holder with the long dimension positioned horizontally.

3. Check posted exposure factors for the dental x-ray unit prior to placing each film packet, and set for the posterior region; adjust as needed for the maxilla and the mandible and for the premolar and molar regions.

4. Place and expose the posterior periapical radiographs in the following order:

1st	right maxillary premolar
2nd	right maxillary molar
3rd	right mandibular premolar
4th	right mandibular molar
5th	left maxillary premolar

6th	left maxillary molar
7th	left mandibular premolar
8th	left mandibular molar

Note: Left-handed radiographers may use this order:

1st	left maxillary premolar
2nd	left maxillary molar
3rd	left mandibular premolar
4th	left mandibular molar
5th	right maxillary premolar
6th	right maxillary molar
7th	right mandibular premolar
8th	right mandibular molar

5. Process the films.

COMPETENCY AND EVALUATION

1. Mount the processed films on the simulated film mounts that follow. Secure with a piece of tape placed along the top edge of the film only, so that the films may be raised slightly, to allow light underneath for ease of viewing. The use of removable transparent tape will allow the film mount page to be used more than once.
   Note: Use the labial mounting method. (See Laboratory Exercise 8, Film Mounting and Radiographic Landmarks, for details.) The raised portion of the embossed dot is toward you (convex) when placing the film onto the page.

2. Place the page with the mounted films taped to it on a view box and evaluate for acceptability. Circle the ✓ where packet placement, vertical angulation, horizontal angulation, and centering were performed correctly, and the ✗ where performed incorrectly. Identify which error was made by placing an ✗ on the corresponding line.

3. Obtain instructor feedback. Identify which step (packet placement, vertical angulation, horizontal angulation, centering) needs improvement.

4. Repeat Part 1 and Part 2 at the direction of your instructor. The film mount page may be copied to accommodate multiple practice attempts to achieve competency.

5. Compare the periapicals taken utilizing the bisecting technique with those taken utilizing the paralleling technique. (See Laboratory Exercise 3, Periapical Radiographs—Paralleling Technique.) Evaluate the images for diagnostic quality differences, and discuss which technique produced the best images. Assess your skills with each of the techniques. Did you find one or the other technique easier to learn? Why? Compare the advantages and disadvantages of the paralleling and the bisecting techniques.

6. Complete the study questions.

NAME _____

Full mouth series A
Part 1: Anterior Periapical Radiographs—Maxilla
Mount Films Below

patient's right   patient's left

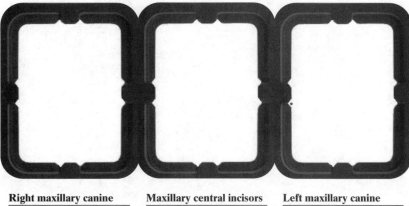

Right maxillary canine		**Maxillary central incisors**		**Left maxillary canine**	
packet placement	✓ ✗	**packet placement**	✓ ✗	**packet placement**	✓ ✗
___ too far anterior		___ too far anterior		___ too far anterior	
___ too far posterior		___ too far posterior		___ too far posterior	
vertical angulation	✓ ✗	**vertical angulation**	✓ ✗	**vertical angulation**	✓ ✗
___ excessive		___ excessive		___ excessive	
___ inadequate		___ inadequate		___ inadequate	
horizontal angulation	✓ ✗	**horizontal angulation**	✓ ✗	**horizontal angulation**	✓ ✗
___ from the mesial		___ from the mesial		___ from the mesial	
___ from the distal		___ from the distal		___ from the distal	
centering the PID	✓ ✗	**centering the PID**	✓ ✗	**centering the PID**	✓ ✗
___ too far anterior		___ too far anterior		___ too far anterior	
___ too far posterior		___ too far posterior		___ too far posterior	
___ too far superior		___ too far superior		___ too far superior	
___ too far inferior		___ too far inferior		___ too far inferior	

Full mouth series A

Part 1: Anterior Periapical Radiographs—Mandible

Mount Films Below

patient's right   patient's left

Right mandibular canine	Mandibular central incisors	Left mandibular canine
packet placement ✓ ✗	**packet placement** ✓ ✗	**packet placement** ✓ ✗
___ too far anterior	___ too far anterior	___ too far anterior
___ too far posterior	___ too far posterior	___ too far posterior
vertical angulation ✓ ✗	**vertical angulation** ✓ ✗	**vertical angulation** ✓ ✗
___ excessive	___ excessive	___ excessive
___ inadequate	___ inadequate	___ inadequate
horizontal angulation ✓ ✗	**horizontal angulation** ✓ ✗	**horizontal angulation** ✓ ✗
___ from the mesial	___ from the mesial	___ from the mesial
___ from the distal	___ from the distal	___ from the distal
centering the PID ✓ ✗	**centering the PID** ✓ ✗	**centering the PID** ✓ ✗
___ too far anterior	___ too far anterior	___ too far anterior
___ too far posterior	___ too far posterior	___ too far posterior
___ too far superior	___ too far superior	___ too far superior
___ too far inferior	___ too far inferior	___ too far inferior

NAME _____

Full mouth series B
Part 1: Anterior Periapical Radiographs—Maxilla
Mount Films Below

patient's right   patient's left

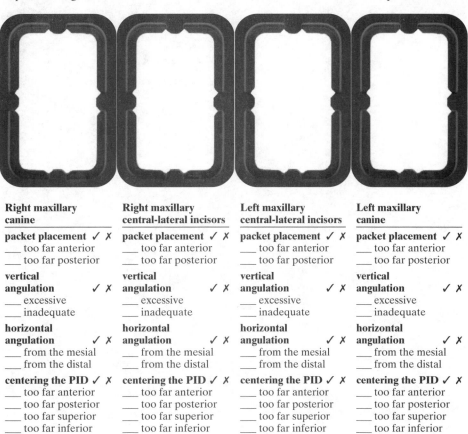

Right maxillary canine	**Right maxillary central-lateral incisors**	**Left maxillary central-lateral incisors**	**Left maxillary canine**
packet placement ✓ ✗	**packet placement** ✓ ✗	**packet placement** ✓ ✗	**packet placement** ✓ ✗
___ too far anterior	___ too far anterior	___ too far anterior	___ too far anterior
___ too far posterior	___ too far posterior	___ too far posterior	___ too far posterior
vertical angulation ✓ ✗	**vertical angulation** ✓ ✗	**vertical angulation** ✓ ✗	**vertical angulation** ✓ ✗
___ excessive	___ excessive	___ excessive	___ excessive
___ inadequate	___ inadequate	___ inadequate	___ inadequate
horizontal angulation ✓ ✗	**horizontal angulation** ✓ ✗	**horizontal angulation** ✓ ✗	**horizontal angulation** ✓ ✗
___ from the mesial	___ from the mesial	___ from the mesial	___ from the mesial
___ from the distal	___ from the distal	___ from the distal	___ from the distal
centering the PID ✓ ✗	**centering the PID** ✓ ✗	**centering the PID** ✓ ✗	**centering the PID** ✓ ✗
___ too far anterior	___ too far anterior	___ too far anterior	___ too far anterior
___ too far posterior	___ too far posterior	___ too far posterior	___ too far posterior
___ too far superior	___ too far superior	___ too far superior	___ too far superior
___ too far inferior	___ too far inferior	___ too far inferior	___ too far inferior

Full mouth series B
Part 1: Anterior Periapical Radiographs—Mandible
Mount Films Below

patient's right   patient's left

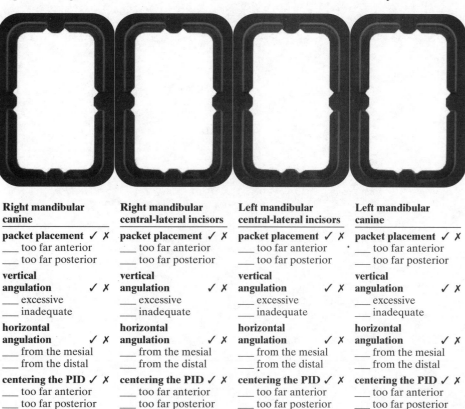

Right mandibular canine	**Right mandibular central-lateral incisors**	**Left mandibular central-lateral incisors**	**Left mandibular canine**
packet placement ✓ ✗	**packet placement** ✓ ✗	**packet placement** ✓ ✗	**packet placement** ✓ ✗
___ too far anterior	___ too far anterior	___ too far anterior	___ too far anterior
___ too far posterior	___ too far posterior	___ too far posterior	___ too far posterior
vertical angulation ✓ ✗	**vertical angulation** ✓ ✗	**vertical angulation** ✓ ✗	**vertical angulation** ✓ ✗
___ excessive	___ excessive	___ excessive	___ excessive
___ inadequate	___ inadequate	___ inadequate	___ inadequate
horizontal angulation ✓ ✗	**horizontal angulation** ✓ ✗	**horizontal angulation** ✓ ✗	**horizontal angulation** ✓ ✗
___ from the mesial	___ from the mesial	___ from the mesial	___ from the mesial
___ from the distal	___ from the distal	___ from the distal	___ from the distal
centering the PID ✓ ✗	**centering the PID** ✓ ✗	**centering the PID** ✓ ✗	**centering the PID** ✓ ✗
___ too far anterior	___ too far anterior	___ too far anterior	___ too far anterior
___ too far posterior	___ too far posterior	___ too far posterior	___ too far posterior
___ too far superior	___ too far superior	___ too far superior	___ too far superior
___ too far inferior	___ too far inferior	___ too far inferior	___ too far inferior

Full mouth series A and B
Part 2: Posterior Periapical Radiographs
Mount Films Below

patient's right side

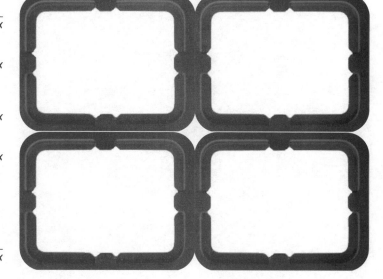

Right maxillary molar

packet placement ✓ ✗
___ too far anterior
___ too far posterior

vertical angulation ✓ ✗
___ excessive
___ inadequate

horizontal angulation ✓ ✗
___ from the mesial
___ from the distal

centering the PID ✓ ✗
___ too far anterior
___ too far posterior
___ too far superior
___ too far inferior

Right mandibular molar

packet placement ✓ ✗
___ too far anterior
___ too far posterior

vertical angulation ✓ ✗
___ excessive
___ inadequate

horizontal angulation ✓ ✗
___ from the mesial
___ from the distal

centering the PID ✓ ✗
___ too far anterior
___ too far posterior
___ too far superior
___ too far inferior

Right maxillary premolar

packet placement ✓ ✗
___ too far anterior
___ too far posterior

vertical angulation ✓ ✗
___ excessive
___ inadequate

horizontal angulation ✓ ✗
___ from the mesial
___ from the distal

centering the PID ✓ ✗
___ too far anterior
___ too far posterior
___ too far superior
___ too far inferior

Right mandibular premolar

packet placement ✓ ✗
___ too far anterior
___ too far posterior

vertical angulation ✓ ✗
___ excessive
___ inadequate

horizontal angulation ✓ ✗
___ from the mesial
___ from the distal

centering the PID ✓ ✗
___ too far anterior
___ too far posterior
___ too far superior
___ too far inferior

Full mouth series A and B
Part 2: Posterior Periapical Radiographs
Mount Films Below

patient's left side

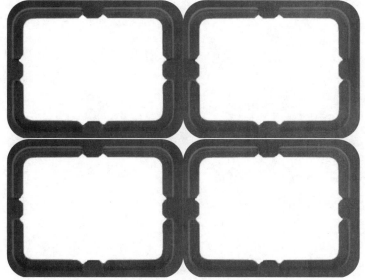

Left maxillary premolar

packet placement ✓ ✗
___ too far anterior
___ too far posterior

vertical angulation ✓ ✗
___ excessive
___ inadequate

**horizontal
angulation** ✓ ✗
___ from the mesial
___ from the distal

centering the PID ✓ ✗
___ too far anterior
___ too far posterior
___ too far superior
___ too far inferior

Left maxillary molar

packet placement ✓ ✗
___ too far anterior
___ too far posterior

vertical angulation ✓ ✗
___ excessive
___ inadequate

**horizontal
angulation** ✓ ✗
___ from the mesial
___ from the distal

centering the PID ✓ ✗
___ too far anterior
___ too far posterior
___ too far superior
___ too far inferior

**Left mandibular
premolar**

packet placement ✓ ✗
___ too far anterior
___ too far posterior

vertical angulation ✓ ✗
___ excessive
___ inadequate

**horizontal
angulation** ✓ ✗
___ from the mesial
___ from the distal

centering the PID ✓ ✗
___ too far anterior
___ too far posterior
___ too far superior
___ too far inferior

**Left mandibular
molar**

packet placement ✓ ✗
___ too far anterior
___ too far posterior

vertical angulation ✓ ✗
___ excessive
___ inadequate

**horizontal
angulation** ✓ ✗
___ from the mesial
___ from the distal

centering the PID ✓ ✗
___ too far anterior
___ too far posterior
___ too far superior
___ too far inferior

I. Bisecting technique
  A. Principle concepts
    1. White unprinted side of the film packet is placed toward the teeth.
    2. The embossed identification dot is positioned away from the area of interest. (Place dot toward the incisal/occlusal edge and away from the apex of the teeth.)
    3. Film packet is placed as close to the teeth as possible. Film will no longer be parallel to the long axis of the tooth.
    4. Central ray of the x-ray beam is directed perpendicular to the imaginary bisector between the film packet and the long axis of the tooth.
    5. Film is held in place by a bite block or other periapical film-holding device.
      a. The bisecting technique evolved before the development of film holders. In the past, the patient's finger or thumb were used to hold the film packet in place in the oral cavity.
      b. It is no longer appropriate to use the patient's finger to hold the film in place because:
        1) The patient may move the film packet out of position.
        2) Excessive pressure from the patient's finger or thumb may bend the film packet, resulting in a distorted image.
        3) The patient's finger will be placed in the path of the primary beam and incur an unnecessary dose of radiation.
        4) The patient may object to placing the fingers in the mouth, or perceive this method as unhygienic and/or unprofessional.
  B. Advantages
    1. Film packet placement may be more comfortable for the patient to tolerate and easier for the operator to achieve. Patients most likely to benefit from the bisecting technique are
      a. Low palatal vault
      b. Tori present
      c. Exaggerated gag reflex
      d. Children (Figure 4.3 ■)
      e. Edentulous
    2. Film packet placement does not require the use of a commercially made film-holding device. Packet may be stabilized with

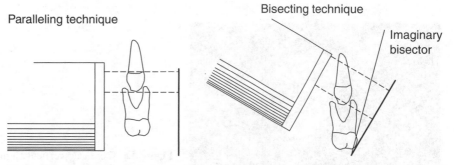

Figure 4.3 Increased vertical angulation used by the bisecting technique has an added advantage of imaging more of the developing permanent teeth of children.

a custom-made holder such as a hemostat (Figure 4.4 ■) or tongue blade.

C. Disadvantages
  1. Increased image distortion inherent to the technique. Slight fore-shortening or elongation of image usually occurs, especially with maxillary multirooted teeth. (Figure 4.5 ■)
  2. Increased incidence of superimposition of adjacent structures, especially of the zygoma over the maxillary posterior teeth roots. (Figure 4.6 ■)
  3. May increase patient radiation exposure, because a short 8" PID is recommended for use with bisecting technique. (Figure 4.7 ■)

II. Periapical radiographic procedure—anterior region
  A. Placement of the film packet—*Full Mouth Series A*. (Figure 4.8 ■) The teeth to be imaged on radiographs exposed utilizing the bisecting technique are the same as those imaged when utilizing the

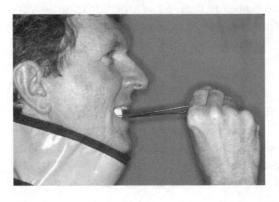

Figure 4.4 Hemostat used as a film-holding device for use with the bisecting technique.

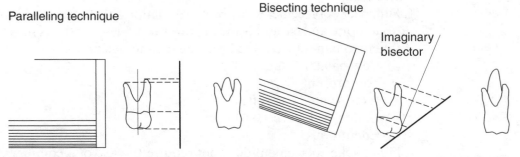

Paralleling technique

Bisecting technique

Imaginary bisector

Figure 4.5 A comparison of palatal root length of the maxillary first molar, when utilizing the paralleling and bisecting techniques.

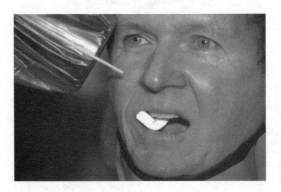

Figure 4.6 Increased vertical angulation for the bisecting technique often superimposes the zygoma over the root apex of the maxillary first molar on the resultant image.

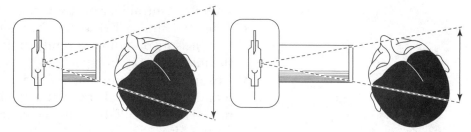

Figure 4.7 A comparison of the diameter of exiting beam of radiation exposure with short and long PIDs.

paralleling technique. The difference between the two techniques is that when utilizing the bisecting technique the film and teeth will not be parallel to each other.

1. Maxillary central incisors periapical radiograph
   a. Align the film packet so that the maxillary central and lateral incisors on both the right and left sides are centered in the middle of the film packet.
   b. Ensure that the film packet is placed such that the entire maxillary central and lateral incisors and the mesial half of both the right and left canines will be recorded on the film.
   c. Place the film packet as close to the central and lateral incisors as possible. Film may contact the lingual surface of the teeth.
2. Maxillary canine periapical radiograph
   a. Align the film packet so that the maxillary canine is centered in the middle of the film packet.
   b. Ensure that the film packet is placed such that the maxillary distal half of the lateral, entire canine, and the mesial half of the first premolar will be recorded on the film.
   c. Place the film packet as close to the canine as possible. Film may contact the lingual surface of the teeth.

Maxillary Central-Lateral Incisors   Maxillary Canine

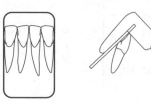

Mandibular Central-Lateral Incisors   Mandibular Canine

Figure 4.8 Full mouth series A—film packet placement for anterior periapical radiographs.

3. Mandibular central incisors periapical radiograph
   a. Align the film packet so that the mandibular central and lateral incisors on both the right and left sides are centered in the middle of the film packet.
   b. Ensure that the film packet is placed such that the entire mandibular central incisors and lateral incisors and the mesial half of both the right and left canines will be recorded on the film.
   c. Place the film packet as close to the central and lateral incisors as possible. Film may contact the lingual surface of the teeth.
4. Mandibular canine periapical radiograph
   a. Align the film packet so that the mandibular canine is centered in the middle of the film packet.
   b. Ensure that the film packet is placed such that the mandibular distal half of the lateral, entire canine, and the mesial half of the first premolar will be recorded on the film.
   c. Place the film packet as close to the canine as possible. Film may contact the lingual surface of the teeth.

B. Placement of the film packet—*Full Mouth Series B* (Figure 4.9 ■)
1. Maxillary central-lateral incisors periapical radiograph
   a. Align the film packet so that the maxillary central and lateral incisors on one side are centered in the middle of the film packet.
   b. Ensure that the film packet is placed such that the maxillary distal half of the central incisor on the opposite side, the entire central and lateral incisors on the side being imaged, and the mesial half of the canine will be recorded on the film.
   c. Place the film packet as close to the central and lateral incisors as possible. Film may contact the lingual surface of the teeth.
2. Maxillary canine periapical radiograph
   a. Align the film packet so that the maxillary canine is centered in the middle of the film packet.
   b. Ensure that the film packet is placed such that the maxillary distal half of the lateral, entire canine, and the mesial half of the first premolar will be recorded on the film.

Maxillary Central-Lateral Incisors

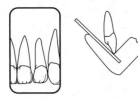

Maxillary Canine

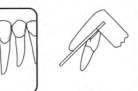

Mandibular Central-Lateral Incisors

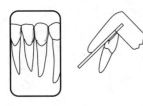

Mandibular Canine

Figure 4.9 Full mouth series B—film packet placement for anterior periapical radiographs.

    c. Place the film packet as close to the canine as possible. Film may contact the lingual surface of the teeth.

  3. Mandibular central-lateral incisors periapical radiograph

    a. Align the film packet so that the mandibular lateral and central incisors on one side are centered in the middle of the film packet.

    b. Ensure that the film packet is placed such that the mandibular distal half of the central incisor on the opposite side, the entire central and lateral incisors on the side being imaged, and the mesial half of the canine will be recorded on the film.

    c. Place the film packet as close to the central and lateral incisors as possible. Film may contact the lingual surface of the teeth.

  4. Mandibular canine periapical radiograph

    a. Align the film packet so that the mandibular canine is centered in the middle of the film packet.

    b. Ensure that the film packet is placed such that the mandibular distal half of the lateral, entire canine, and the mesial half of the first premolar will be recorded on the film.

    c. Place the film packet as close to the canine as possible. Film may contact the lingual surface of the teeth.

III. Periapical radiographic procedure—posterior region

  A. Placement of the film packet—*Same for all full mouth series configurations* (Figure 4.10 ■)

    1. Maxillary premolar periapical radiograph

     a. Align the mesial edge of the film packet far enough forward to line up behind the middle of the maxillary canine.

     b. Ensure that the film packet is placed such that the maxillary distal half of the canine, first and second premolars, first molar and mesial half of the second molar will be recorded on the film.

     c. Place the film packet as close to the premolars as possible. Film may contact the lingual surface of the teeth.

    2. Maxillary molar periapical radiograph

     a. Align the mesial edge of the film packet behind the middle of the maxillary second premolar.

     b. Ensure that the film packet is placed such that the maxillary distal half of the second premolar, and first, second, and third molar will be recorded on the film.

Maxillary Premolar   Maxillary Molar

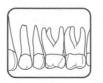 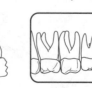

Mandibular Premolar   Mandibular Molar

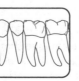

Figure 4.10 Full mouth series A, B, C, D—film packet placement for posterior periapical radiographs.

    c. Place the film packet as close to the molars as possible. Film may contact the lingual surface of the teeth.

  3. Mandibular premolar periapical radiograph

    a. Align the mesial edge of the film packet far enough forward to line up behind the middle of the mandibular canine.

    b. Ensure that the film packet is placed such that the mandibular distal half of the canine, first and second premolars, first molar, and mesial half of the second molar will be recorded on the film.

    c. Place the film packet as close to the premolars as possible. Film may contact the lingual surface of the teeth.

  4. Mandibular molar periapical radiograph

    a. Align the mesial edge of the film packet behind the middle of the mandibular second premolar.

    b. Ensure that the film packet is placed such that the mandibular distal half of the second premolar, and first, second, and third molar will be recorded on the film.

    c. Place the film packet as close to the molars as possible. Film may contact the lingual surface of the teeth.

IV. Vertical Angulation

  A. Generally the vertical angulation will be increased over the vertical angulation normally used when there is a parallel film packet placement. To compensate for the "flatter" placement of the film packet when utilizing the bisecting technique, the vertical angulation is increased.

  B. Direct the x-ray beam to intersect the imaginary bisector between the film packet plane and the plane of the long axis of the tooth perpendicularly. (Figure 4.11 ■) As a visual aid in estimating the imaginary bisector and determining the correct vertical angulation, align the vertical angulation of the PID perpendicular to the film. Make a mental note of this angle. Then realign the PID so that it is now perpendicular to the tooth, and note this angle. Finally, realign the vertical angle of the PID halfway between the two points noted. Reposition the PID perpendicular to the film, then perpendicular to the tooth several times, until you can make an accurate judgment of the halfway point. (Figures 4.12 ■ and 4.13 ■) Another technique to help estimate the imaginary bisector

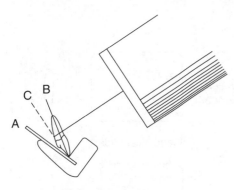

A = Film plane
B = Long axis of the tooth
C = Imaginary bisector

Figure 4.11 Vertical angulation for periapical radiographs using the bisecting technique should be such that the beam will intersect the imaginary bisector between the plane of the film packet and the plane of the tooth perpendicularly in the vertical dimension.

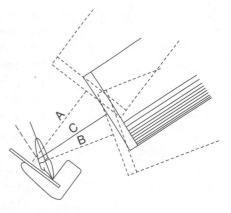

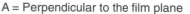

A = Perpendicular to the film plane
B = Perpendicular to the long axis of the tooth
C = Perpendicular to the imaginary bisector

Figure 4.12 Use the two visible planes, the film packet, and the long axis of the tooth to estimate the invisible imaginary bisector.

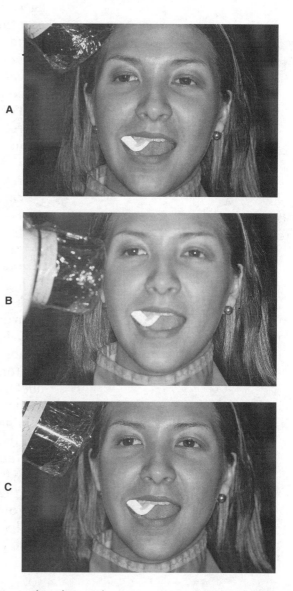

Figure 4.13 (A) PID is directed perpendicular to the film plane. **(B)** PID is directed perpendicular to the long axes of the teeth. **(C)** PID is directed perpendicular to the imaginary bisector between these two planes.

location is to align the PID perpendicular to the film packet plane and note the vertical angulation degrees on the tube head. Realign the PID perpendicular to the long axis of the tooth, and note this angle on the tube head. Add or subtract to locate the halfway point between these two angles and realign the PID at this angle for the exposure.

C. If the patient's head is correctly and precisely positioned, predetermined vertical angulations may be used (Table 4.1).

V. Horizontal Angulation

A. Horizontal angulation of the x-ray beam is determined in the same manner as when utilizing the paralleling technique.

1. Determine the side-to-side placement of the PID.

2. Align the PID such that the central ray of the x-ray beam will intersect the film perpendicularly on the horizontal plane. Perpendicular alignment of the beam can be achieved either of two ways:

a. Direct the central ray of the x-ray beam through a predetermined interproximal space or directly at the tooth being imaged. Examine the contact points of the patient's teeth to determine the correct horizontal angulation. Use the following guidelines (see Figure 3.10):

1) For the central incisors periapical radiograph, direct the central ray of the x-ray beam between the right and left central incisors.

2) For the central-lateral incisors periapical radiograph, direct the central ray of the x-ray beam between the central incisor and lateral incisor.

3) For the canine periapical radiograph, direct the central ray of the x-ray beam directly at the middle of the canine.

4) For the premolar periapical radiograph, direct the central ray between the first and second premolars.

5) For the molar periapical radiograph, direct the central ray between the first and second molars.

b. Using the open end of the PID as the reference point, align such that the open end of the PID is parallel to the film in the horizontal plane. Visualizing the horizontal placement of the PID is easily achieved by placing a tongue blade across the open end and rotating the tube head horizontally until the tongue blade and, hence, the open end of the PID is parallel to the film. (Figure 4.14 ■)

VI. Centering the x-ray beam over the film packet

A. Determining the location of the film packet is slightly more difficult with the bisecting technique. Because of the "flatter" placement of the film packet, the radiographer must be skilled in estimating the direction the x-ray beam will travel once it has traveled past the end of the PID. Use any part of the film holder that is visible outside the mouth as an indication of where the film packet is located.

B. Direct the central rays of the x-ray beam toward the center of the film.

C. Using the Stabe® film holder as a reference point, align the PID directly over the film packet. The film will usually be centered in the diameter of the PID when the edge of the PID is positioned 1/4″ beyond the holder edge. (Figure 4.15 ■) Correct placement of the PID can be achieved by placing the tongue blade as an extension of the PID. No part of the film packet should be visible beyond the diameter of the PID when extending the tongue blade. (Figure 4.16 ■)

D. If the patient's head is correctly and precisely positioned, predetermined points of entry may be used (Table 4.1).

VII. Errors

A. Packet placement error
1. This occurs when the film packet is not placed correctly intraorally.
2. Packet placement errors occur in the same manner as when utilizing the paralleling technique. (Figures 3.14 and 3.15)

B. Vertical angulation error
1. Occurs when the up-and-down angle of the PID is not set such that the x-ray beam intersects the imaginary bisector perpendicularly in the vertical plane
2. Results in an elongation or foreshortening error

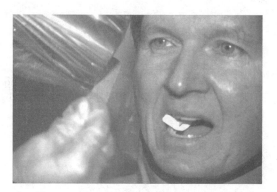

Figure 4.14 Use of a tongue blade acts as a visual aid in determining the correct horizontal angulation.

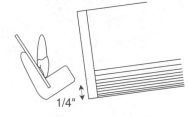

Figure 4.15 PID will be centered over the film packet when the edge of the PID is aligned into position 1/4″ below the Stabe® film holder bite block.

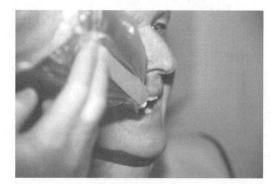

Figure 4.16 Use of a tongue blade acts as a visual aid in determining centering of the x-ray beam over the film packet.

3. Excessive vertical angulation when utilizing the bisecting technique results in a foreshortened image (Figure 4.17 ■)
4. Inadequate vertical angulation when utilizing the bisecting technique results in an elongated image (Figure 4.18 ■)

C. Horizontal angulation error
1. This occurs when the side-to-side angulation of the PID is not set such that the beam will intersect with the film perpendicularly.
2. Horizontal angulation errors occur in the same manner as when utilizing the paralleling technique. (See Figures 3.18 and 3.19)

D. Centering the x-ray beam over the film error
1. This occurs when the PID is not placed directly over the film packet.
2. Centering the x-ray beam over the film results in cone-cut errors in the same manner as when utilizing the paralleling technique. (See Figures 3.20, 3.21, 3.22, and 3.23.)

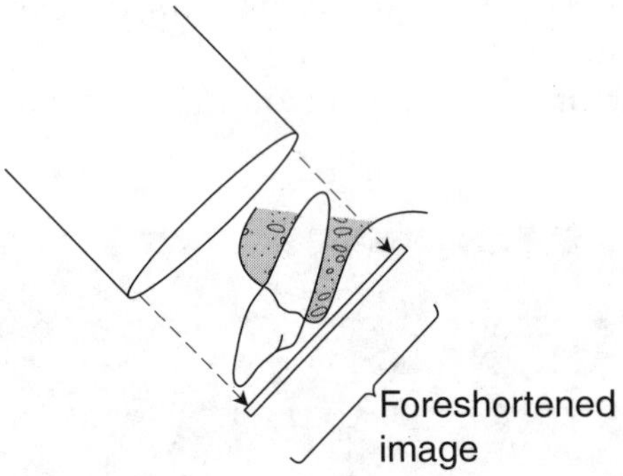

Foreshortened image

Figure 4.17 When utilizing the bisecting technique, excessive vertical angulation results in foreshortening distortion of the image.

Elongated image

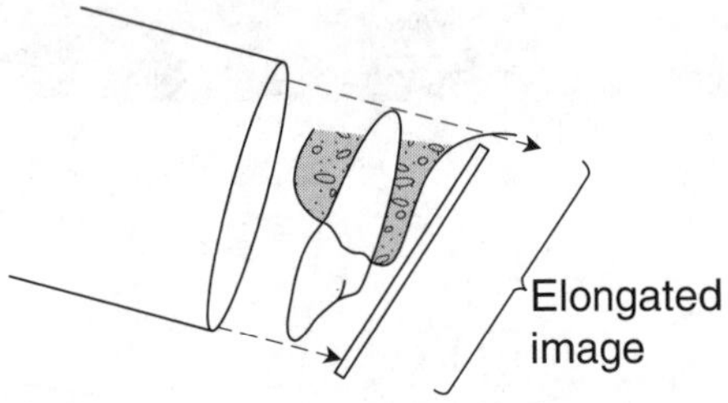

Figure 4.18 When utilizing the bisecting technique, inadequate vertical angulation results in elongation distortion of the image.

BIBLIOGRAPHY

Johnson, ON, Thomson, EM. *Essentials of Dental Radiography for Dental Assistants and Hygienists,* 8th ed. Upper Saddle River, NJ: Prentice Hall; 2007: 137–1 9.

Thomson, EM. Dental radiographs for the child client. *Dental Hygienist News,* 1993; 6: 19–20, 24.

White, SC, Pharoah, MJ. *Oral Radiology Principles and Interpretation,* 5th ed. St. Louis, MO. Elsevier; 2004: 125.

1. Through which interproximal space should the central x-ray beam be directed when exposing a maxillary *premolar* periapical radiograph to achieve accurate horizontal angulation?
   A. Between the canine and the first premolar
   B. Between the first premolar and the second premolar
   C. Between the second premolar and the first molar
   D. Between the first molar and the second molar
   E. Between the second molar and the third molar

2. Through which interproximal space should the central x-ray beam be directed when exposing a mandibular *molar* periapical radiograph to achieve accurate horizontal angulation?
   A. Between the canine and the first premolar
   B. Between the first premolar and the second premolar
   C. Between the second premolar and the first molar
   D. Between the first molar and the second molar
   E. Between the second molar and the third molar

3. A maxillary lateral-canine periapical radiograph did not image the interproximal contact area between the lateral incisor and the central incisor results from an error made in which of the following?
   A. Packet placement
   B. Vertical angulation
   C. Horizontal angulation
   D. Centering the x-ray beam

4. Referring to question 3, which of the following would correct this error?
   A. Position the film packet more anteriorly.
   B. Decrease vertical angulation.
   C. Shift the horizontal angulation toward the distal.
   D. Direct the PID more superiorly.

5. Elongated images results from an error made in which of the following?
   A. Packet placement
   B. Vertical angulation
   C. Horizontal angulation
   D. Centering the x-ray beam

6. Referring to question 5, which of the following would correct this error?
   A. Place the film packet farther away from the teeth
   B. Increase the vertical angulation
   C. Shift the horizontal angulation toward the mesial
   D. Direct the PID more inferiorly

7. Foreshortened images results from an error made in which of the following?
   A. Packet placement
   B. Vertical angulation
   C. Horizontal angulation
   D. Centering the x-ray beam

8. Referring to question 7, which of the following would correct this error?
   A. Place the film packet closer to the teeth.
   B. Decrease the vertical angulation.
   C. Shift the horizontal angulation toward the distal.
   D. Direct the PID more posteriorly.

9. A molar periapical radiograph that is undiagnostic due to overlapped interproximal areas is the result of incorrect:
   A. Packet placement
   B. Vertical angulation
   C. Horizontal angulation
   D. Centering the x-ray beam

10. Compare and contrast the paralleling and the bisecting techniques. List the advantages and disadvantages of each. Indicate under what conditions and circumstances you would utilize the paralleling technique; the bisecting technique.

_____

_____

_____

_____

_____

_____

_____

_____

_____

_____

Radiographic Techniques with Supplemental Film Holders

INTRODUCTION

There is a wide variety of commercially made film-holding devices available. (Figure 5.1 ■) There are film holders specifically designed to expose bitewing radiographs and others for exposing peripical radiographs. Most periapical radiographic film holders are further divided into paralleling or bisecting technique instruments. Some can be modified for use with both techniques. Many manufactures produce a "set" of film holders to be used in conjunction with each other in obtaining a full mouth series of radiographs. It may not be practical or possible to introduce every film-holding device currently on the market, and new products continue to be introduced. However, with a thorough understanding of film packet placement and a mastery of the basic skills required to determine appropriate angulation, the radiographer should be prepared to use any film holder to achieve accurate imagery. Developing the basic intraoral radiography techniques using simple holders, such as the bitewing stick-on tab and the one-piece construction of the polystyrene Stabe® (Dentsply Rinn) introduced in this manual, the radiographer will be prepared to transfer these skills to most any other film holder.

This laboratory exercise will utilize problem-based learning to challenge the student to make decisions regarding the use of the paralleling and the bisecting techniques and to apply basic knowledge of film holder

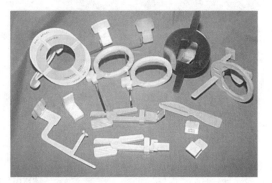

Figure 5.1 A sample of some of the film holders being used in practice. Top, left to right: VIP-2 (UPRAD Corporation www.uprad.com); XCP and BAI (Dentsply Rinn Corporation www.rinncorp.com); Precision-Safe™ (Masel www.maselortho.com); In-trax (previously manufactured by Flow X-Ray Corporation www.flowxray.com). Bottom, left to right: Uni-Bite, Stabe, and Snap-A-Ray (Dentsply Rinn Corporation www.rinncorp.com); Sure Shot (previously available from Jermyn Company, Rochester, NY); self adhesive bitewing tabs and bitewing loops (Flow X-Ray Corporation www.flowxray.com)

design when confronted with an unfamiliar film-holding device. The film holders used in this laboratory exercise are suggestions. The student may be directed to work through the activities using products available at his/her institution. This exercise suggests exposing one-half of the mouth at a time with different film-holding devices. The number and size of films exposed for this exercise remains the same as those recommended in Laboratory Exercises 3 and 4.

OBJECTIVES

Following completion of this lab activity, you will be able to:

1. Identify whether a film holder can be used to expose bitewing or periapcial radiographs.

2. Identify which technique, paralleling or bisecting, should be utilized when confronted with an unfamiliar film-holding device.

3. Correctly place and expose anterior and posterior periapical and bitewing radiographs when given an unfamiliar film-holding device.

4. Demonstrate proficiency in placing, exposing, and processing anterior and posterior periapical and bitewing radiographs using a variety of film-holding devices.

5. List the advantages and disadvantages of various film-holding devices.

MATERIALS

Teaching manikin or skull

Lead (or lead-equivalent) apron with thyroid collar

Size #1 and size #2 radiographic films

Supplemental film holders

Film holders illustrated in this laboratory exercise:

- XCP Instrument Kit available from Dentsply Rinn (www.rinncorp.com) (Figure 5.2 ■)

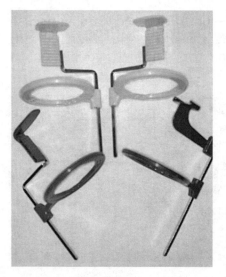

Figure 5.2 XCP Intrument Kit. Note the external aiming ring.

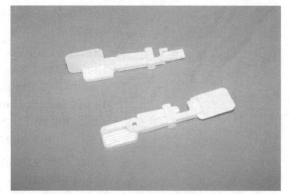

Figure 5.3 Snap-A-Ray film holder demonstrating film packet assembly for posterior (top) and anterior (bottom) periapical radiographs.

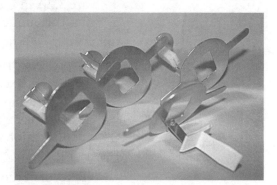

Figure 5.4 Precision Safe™ film holders. Note the external collimator for reducing patient radiation exposure.

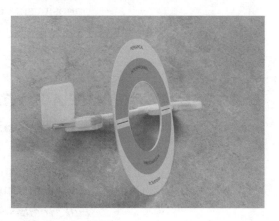

Figure 5.5 VIP-2 System film holder. Note the labeled external aiming device. (Courtesy of UPRAD Corporation.)

- Snap-A-Ray available from Dentsply Rinn (www.rinncorp.com) (Figure 5.3 ■)
- Precision-Safe™ Instrument available from Masel (www.maselortho.com) (Figure 5.4 ■)
- VIP-2 System available from UPRAD Corporation (www.uprad.com) (Figure 5.5 ■)

View box

PREPARATION

1. Study the chapter outline to prepare for this laboratory exercise. An understanding of the material presented in the outline is required to complete this activity.

2. Instructor demonstration may enhance knowledge of the laboratory exercise.

3. Prepare radiology operatory. Set up teaching manikin or skull. Ensure that correct "patient" positioning is achieved. To image the maxilla, ensure that the maxillary occlusal plane is parallel to the floor; to image the mandible, ensure that the mandibular occlusal plane is parallel to the floor and the midsagittal plane must be perpendicular to the floor for both maxillary and mandibular exposures.

4. Place lead apron (or lead-equivalent barrier) and thyroid collar over the "patient."

5. This exercise will use the full mouth series configuration shown in Figure 3.2A in Laboratory Exercise 3, Periapical Radiographs—Paralleling Technique.

6. Obtain the film holders to be used for this exercise.

7. Orient the film packet in the film holder so that the embossed identification dot will be placed away from the apices of the teeth when exposing periapical radiographs. If the film holder has a film retention groove, place the "dot in the slot" of the film holder to position the identification dot of the film packet toward the incisal/occlusal edges of the teeth.

8. Take all of the exposures, bitewings and periapicals, on one side of the mouth using one of the film holders. Take all of the exposures on the opposite side of the mouth with a different film holder.

9. Check posted exposure settings for the dental x-ray unit prior to placing each film packet and appropriately.

LABORATORY EXERCISE ACTIVITIES

Part 1: Periapical and Bitewing Radiographs Using the XCP Film Holder

1. Expose all radiographs on the patient's right side using the XCP film holding instruments. Expose the radiographs in the following order:

   Full Mouth Series A

1st	maxillary central incisors periapical
2nd	right maxillary canine periapical
3rd	mandibular central incisors periapical
4th	right mandibular canine periapical
5th	right maxillary premolar periapical
6th	right maxillary molar periapical
7th	right mandibular premolar periapical
8th	right mandibular molar periapical
9th	right premolar bitewing
10th	right molar bitewing

2. Process the films.

Part 2: Periapical and Bitewing Radiographs Using the Snap-A-Ray Film Holder

1. Expose all radiographs on the patient's left side using the Snap-A-Ray film holding instrument. Expose the radiographs in the following order:

Full Mouth Series A

1st left maxillary canine periapical

2nd left mandibular canine periapical

3rd left maxillary premolar periapical

4th left maxillary molar periapical

5th left mandibular premolar periapical

6th left mandibular molar periapical

7th left premolar bitewing

8th left molar bitewing

2. Process the films.

Part 3: Periapical and Bitewing Radiographs Using the Precision-Safe™ Film Holder

1. Expose all radiographs on the patient's right side using the Precision-Safe™ film holding instruments. Expose the radiographs in the following order:

Full Mouth Series A

1st maxillary central incisors periapical

2nd right maxillary canine periapical

3rd mandibular central incisors periapical

4th right mandibular canine periapical

5th right maxillary premolar periapical

6th right maxillary molar periapical

7th right mandibular premolar periapical

8th right mandibular molar periapical

9th right premolar bitewing

10th right molar bitewing

2. Process the films.

Part 4: Periapical and Bitewing Radiographs Using the VIP-2 System Film Holder

1. Expose all radiographs on the patient's left side using the VIP-2™ film holding instruments. Expose the radiographs in the following order:

Full Mouth Series A

1st left maxillary canine periapical

2nd left mandibular canine periapical

3rd left maxillary premolar periapical

4th left maxillary molar periapical

5th left mandibular premolar periapical

6th left mandibular molar periapical

7th left premolar bitewing

8th left molar bitewing

2. Process the films.

COMPETENCY AND EVALUATION

1. Mount the processed films on the simulated film mounts that follow. Secure with a piece of tape placed along the top edge of the film only, so that the films may be raised slightly, to allow light underneath for ease of viewing. The use of removable transparent tape will allow the film mount page to be used more than once.

   Note: Use the labial mounting method. (See Laboratory Exercise 8, Film Mounting and Radiographic Landmarks, for details.) The raised portion of the embossed dot is toward you (convex) when placing the film onto the page.

2. Place the page with the mounted films taped to it on a view box and evaluate for acceptability. Circle the ✓ where packet placement, vertical angulation, horizontal angulation, and centering were performed correctly, and the ✗ where performed incorrectly. Identify which error was made by placing an ✗ on the corresponding line.

3. Obtain instructor feedback. Identify which step (packet placement, vertical angulation, horizontal angulation, centering) needs improvement.

4. Repeat the exercise with other film holders at the direction of your instructor. The film mount page may be copied to accommodate multiple practice attempts to achieve competency.

5. Compare the radiographs taken with each of the 4 holders. Evaluate the images for diagnostic quality differences, and discuss which holders seemed easiest/most difficult to work with. Were there differences in the ease of placement? Were any of the devices more difficult to figure out how to use? What criteria did you use to decide which holders should be used to expose bitewing radiographs and which holders would be used to expose periapical radiographs? Assess your skills with each of the holders. List the advantages and disadvantages of each of the holders you worked with.

6. Complete the study questions.

NAME _____

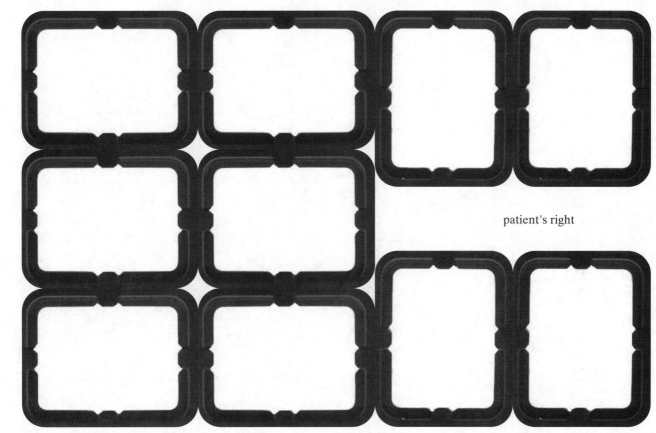

patient's right

Part 1: Periapical and Bitewing Radiographs Using the XCP Film Holder
Evaluation of Radiographs

Right maxillary molar

packet placement ✓ X
___ too far anterior
___ too far posterior

vertical
angulation ✓ X
___ excessive
___ inadequate

horizontal
angulation ✓ X
___ from the mesial
___ from the distal

centering the PID ✓ X
___ too far anterior
___ too far posterior
___ too far superior
___ too far inferior

Right maxillary premolar

packet placement ✓ X
___ too far anterior
___ too far posterior

vertical
angulation ✓ X
___ excessive
___ inadequate

horizontal
angulation ✓ X
___ from the mesial
___ from the distal

centering the PID ✓ X
___ too far anterior
___ too far posterior
___ too far superior
___ too far inferior

Right maxillary canine

packet placement ✓ X
___ too far anterior
___ too far posterior

vertical
angulation ✓ X
___ excessive
___ inadequate

horizontal
angulation ✓ X
___ from the mesial
___ from the distal

centering the PID ✓ X
___ too far anterior
___ too far posterior
___ too far superior
___ too far inferior

Maxillary central incisors

packet placement ✓ X
___ too far anterior
___ too far posterior

vertical
angulation ✓ X
___ excessive
___ inadequate

horizontal
angulation ✓ X
___ from the mesial
___ from the distal

centering the PID ✓ X
___ too far anterior
___ too far posterior
___ too far superior
___ too far inferior

Right molar bitewing

packet placement ✓ X
___ too far anterior
___ too far posterior

vertical
angulation ✓ X
___ excessive
___ inadequate

horizontal
angulation ✓ X
___ from the mesial
___ from the distal

centering the PID ✓ X
___ too far anterior
___ too far posterior
___ too far superior
___ too far inferior

Right premolar bitewing

packet placement ✓ X
___ too far anterior
___ too far posterior

vertical
angulation ✓ X
___ excessive
___ inadequate

horizontal
angulation ✓ X
___ from the mesial
___ from the distal

centering the PID ✓ X
___ too far anterior
___ too far posterior
___ too far superior
___ too far inferior

Right mandibular molar

packet placement ✓ X
___ too far anterior
___ too far posterior

vertical
angulation ✓ X
___ excessive
___ inadequate

horizontal
angulation ✓ X
___ from the mesial
___ from the distal

centering the PID ✓ X
___ too far anterior
___ too far posterior
___ too far superior
___ too far inferior

Right mandibular premolar

packet placement ✓ X
___ too far anterior
___ too far posterior

vertical
angulation ✓ X
___ excessive
___ inadequate

horizontal
angulation ✓ X
___ from the mesial
___ from the distal

centering the PID ✓ X
___ too far anterior
___ too far posterior
___ too far superior
___ too far inferior

Right mandibular canine

packet placement ✓ X
___ too far anterior
___ too far posterior

vertical
angulation ✓ X
___ excessive
___ inadequate

horizontal
angulation ✓ X
___ from the mesial
___ from the distal

centering the PID ✓ X
___ too far anterior
___ too far posterior
___ too far superior
___ too far inferior

Mandibular central incisors

packet placement ✓ X
___ too far anterior
___ too far posterior

vertical
angulation ✓ X
___ excessive
___ inadequate

horizontal
angulation ✓ X
___ from the mesial
___ from the distal

centering the PID ✓ X
___ too far anterior
___ too far posterior
___ too far superior
___ too far inferior

Part 2: Periapical and Bitewing Radiographs Using the Snap-A-Ray Film Holder
Mount Films Below

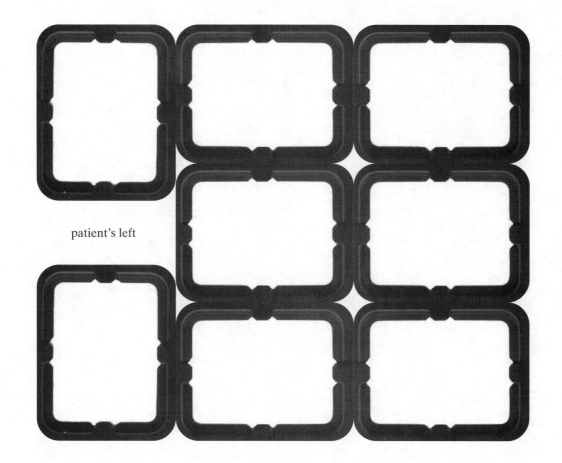

patient's left

Part 2: Periapical and Bitewing Radiographs Using the Snap-A-Ray Film Holder
Evaluation of Radiographs

Left maxillary canine

packet placement ✓ ✗
___ too far anterior
___ too far posterior

vertical angulation ✓ ✗
___ excessive
___ inadequate

horizontal angulation ✓ ✗
___ from the mesial
___ from the distal

centering the PID ✓ ✗
___ too far anterior
___ too far posterior
___ too far superior
___ too far inferior

Left maxillary premolar

packet placement ✓ ✗
___ too far anterior
___ too far posterior

vertical angulation ✓ ✗
___ excessive
___ inadequate

horizontal angulation ✓ ✗
___ from the mesial
___ from the distal

centering the PID ✓ ✗
___ too far anterior
___ too far posterior
___ too far superior
___ too far inferior

Left maxillary molar

packet placement ✓ ✗
___ too far anterior
___ too far posterior

vertical angulation ✓ ✗
___ excessive
___ inadequate

horizontal angulation ✓ ✗
___ from the mesial
___ from the distal

centering the PID ✓ ✗
___ too far anterior
___ too far posterior
___ too far superior
___ too far inferior

Left premolar bitewing

packet placement ✓ ✗
___ too far anterior
___ too far posterior

vertical angulation ✓ ✗
___ excessive
___ inadequate

horizontal angulation ✓ ✗
___ from the mesial
___ from the distal

centering the PID ✓ ✗
___ too far anterior
___ too far posterior
___ too far superior
___ too far inferior

Left molar bitewing

packet placement ✓ ✗
___ too far anterior
___ too far posterior

vertical angulation ✓ ✗
___ excessive
___ inadequate

horizontal angulation ✓ ✗
___ from the mesial
___ from the distal

centering the PID ✓ ✗
___ too far anterior
___ too far posterior
___ too far superior
___ too far inferior

Left mandibular canine

packet placement ✓ ✗
___ too far anterior
___ too far posterior

vertical angulation ✓ ✗
___ excessive
___ inadequate

horizontal angulation ✓ ✗
___ from the mesial
___ from the distal

centering the PID ✓ ✗
___ too far anterior
___ too far posterior
___ too far superior
___ too far inferior

Left mandibular premolar

packet placement ✓ ✗
___ too far anterior
___ too far posterior

vertical angulation ✓ ✗
___ excessive
___ inadequate

horizontal angulation ✓ ✗
___ from the mesial
___ from the distal

centering the PID ✓ ✗
___ too far anterior
___ too far posterior
___ too far superior
___ too far inferior

Left mandibular molar

packet placement ✓ ✗
___ too far anterior
___ too far posterior

vertical angulation ✓ ✗
___ excessive
___ inadequate

horizontal angulation ✓ ✗
___ from the mesial
___ from the distal

centering the PID ✓ ✗
___ too far anterior
___ too far posterior
___ too far superior
___ too far inferior

Part 3: Periapical and Bitewing Radiographs Using the Precision-Safe™ Film Holder
Mount Films Below

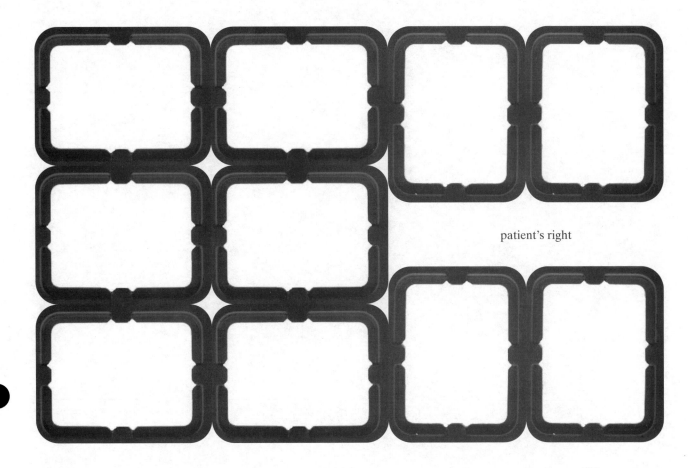

patient's right

Part 3: Periapical and Bitewing Radiographs Using the Precision-Safe™ Film Holder
Evaluation of Radiographs

Right maxillary molar

packet placement ✓ ✗
___ too far anterior
___ too far posterior

vertical angulation ✓ ✗
___ excessive
___ inadequate

horizontal angulation ✓ ✗
___ from the mesial
___ from the distal

centering the PID ✓ ✗
___ too far anterior
___ too far posterior
___ too far superior
___ too far inferior

Right maxillary premolar

packet placement ✓ ✗
___ too far anterior
___ too far posterior

vertical angulation ✓ ✗
___ excessive
___ inadequate

horizontal angulation ✓ ✗
___ from the mesial
___ from the distal

centering the PID ✓ ✗
___ too far anterior
___ too far posterior
___ too far superior
___ too far inferior

Right maxillary canine

packet placement ✓ ✗
___ too far anterior
___ too far posterior

vertical angulation ✓ ✗
___ excessive
___ inadequate

horizontal angulation ✓ ✗
___ from the mesial
___ from the distal

centering the PID ✓ ✗
___ too far anterior
___ too far posterior
___ too far superior
___ too far inferior

Maxillary central incisors

packet placement ✓ ✗
___ too far anterior
___ too far posterior

vertical angulation ✓ ✗
___ excessive
___ inadequate

horizontal angulation ✓ ✗
___ from the mesial
___ from the distal

centering the PID ✓ ✗
___ too far anterior
___ too far posterior
___ too far superior
___ too far inferior

Right molar bitewing

packet placement ✓ ✗
___ too far anterior
___ too far posterior

vertical angulation ✓ ✗
___ excessive
___ inadequate

horizontal angulation ✓ ✗
___ from the mesial
___ from the distal

centering the PID ✓ ✗
___ too far anterior
___ too far posterior
___ too far superior
___ too far inferior

Right premolar bitewing

packet placement ✓ ✗
___ too far anterior
___ too far posterior

vertical angulation ✓ ✗
___ excessive
___ inadequate

horizontal angulation ✓ ✗
___ from the mesial
___ from the distal

centering the PID ✓ ✗
___ too far anterior
___ too far posterior
___ too far superior
___ too far inferior

Right mandibular molar

packet placement ✓ ✗
___ too far anterior
___ too far posterior

vertical angulation ✓ ✗
___ excessive
___ inadequate

horizontal angulation ✓ ✗
___ from the mesial
___ from the distal

centering the PID ✓ ✗
___ too far anterior
___ too far posterior
___ too far superior
___ too far inferior

Right mandibular premolar

packet placement ✓ ✗
___ too far anterior
___ too far posterior

vertical angulation ✓ ✗
___ excessive
___ inadequate

horizontal angulation ✓ ✗
___ from the mesial
___ from the distal

centering the PID ✓ ✗
___ too far anterior
___ too far posterior
___ too far superior
___ too far inferior

Right mandibular canine

packet placement ✓ ✗
___ too far anterior
___ too far posterior

vertical angulation ✓ ✗
___ excessive
___ inadequate

horizontal angulation ✓ ✗
___ from the mesial
___ from the distal

centering the PID ✓ ✗
___ too far anterior
___ too far posterior
___ too far superior
___ too far inferior

Mandibular central incisors

packet placement ✓ ✗
___ too far anterior
___ too far posterior

vertical angulation ✓ ✗
___ excessive
___ inadequate

horizontal angulation ✓ ✗
___ from the mesial
___ from the distal

centering the PID ✓ ✗
___ too far anterior
___ too far posterior
___ too far superior
___ too far inferior

Part 4: Periapical and Bitewing Radiographs Using the VIP-2 Film Holder
Mount Films Below

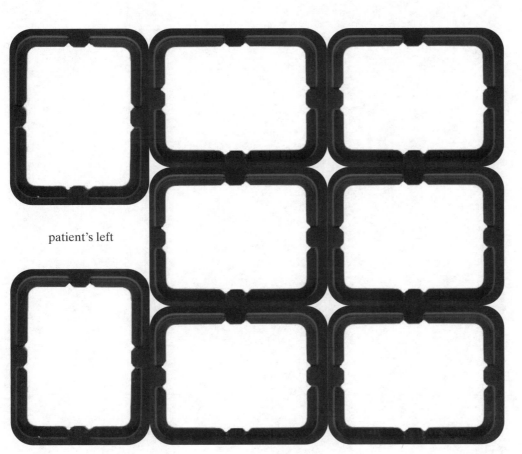

patient's left

Part 4: Periapical and Bitewing Radiographs Using the VIP-2 Film Holder
Evaluation of Radiographs

**Left maxillary
canine** _____

packet placement ✓ ✗
___ too far anterior
___ too far posterior

**vertical
angulation** ✓ ✗
___ excessive
___ inadequate

**horizontal
angulation** ✓ ✗
___ from the mesial
___ from the distal

centering the PID ✓ ✗
___ too far anterior
___ too far posterior
___ too far superior
___ too far inferior

**Left maxillary
premolar** _____

packet placement ✓ ✗
___ too far anterior
___ too far posterior

**vertical
angulation** ✓ ✗
___ excessive
___ inadequate

**horizontal
angulation** ✓ ✗
___ from the mesial
___ from the distal

centering the PID ✓ ✗
___ too far anterior
___ too far posterior
___ too far superior
___ too far inferior

**Left maxillary
molar** _____

packet placement ✓ ✗
___ too far anterior
___ too far posterior

**vertical
angulation** ✓ ✗
___ excessive
___ inadequate

**horizontal
angulation** ✓ ✗
___ from the mesial
___ from the distal

centering the PID ✓ ✗
___ too far anterior
___ too far posterior
___ too far superior
___ too far inferior

**Left premolar
bitewing** _____

packet placement ✓ ✗
___ too far anterior
___ too far posterior

**vertical
angulation** ✓ ✗
___ excessive
___ inadequate

**horizontal
angulation** ✓ ✗
___ from the mesial
___ from the distal

centering the PID ✓ ✗
___ too far anterior
___ too far posterior
___ too far superior
___ too far inferior

**Left molar
bitewing** _____

packet placement ✓ ✗
___ too far anterior
___ too far posterior

**vertical
angulation** ✓ ✗
___ excessive
___ inadequate

**horizontal
angulation** ✓ ✗
___ from the mesial
___ from the distal

centering the PID ✓ ✗
___ too far anterior
___ too far posterior
___ too far superior
___ too far inferior

**Left mandibular
canine** _____

packet placement ✓ ✗
___ too far anterior
___ too far posterior

**vertical
angulation** ✓ ✗
___ excessive
___ inadequate

**horizontal
angulation** ✓ ✗
___ from the mesial
___ from the distal

centering the PID ✓ ✗
___ too far anterior
___ too far posterior
___ too far superior
___ too far inferior

**Left mandibular
premolar** _____

packet placement ✓ ✗
___ too far anterior
___ too far posterior

**vertical
angulation** ✓ ✗
___ excessive
___ inadequate

**horizontal
angulation** ✓ ✗
___ from the mesial
___ from the distal

centering the PID ✓ ✗
___ too far anterior
___ too far posterior
___ too far superior
___ too far inferior

**Left mandibular
molar** _____

packet placement ✓ ✗
___ too far anterior
___ too far posterior

**vertical
angulation** ✓ ✗
___ excessive
___ inadequate

**horizontal
angulation** ✓ ✗
___ from the mesial
___ from the distal

centering the PID ✓ ✗
___ too far anterior
___ too far posterior
___ too far superior
___ too far inferior

I. Film-holding instruments
   A. Prior to the development of film holders, the patient's finger or thumb were used to hold the film packet in place in the oral cavity. It is no longer appropriate to use the patient's finger or thumb to hold the film in place because:
      1. Increased patient instruction and cooperation is required.
      2. It is highly unlikely that the patient will be able to position the film parallel to the teeth.
      3. The patient may move the film packet out of position.
      4. Excessive pressure from the patient's finger or thumb may bend the film packet, resulting in a distorted image.
      5. The patient's finger will be placed in the path of the primary beam and incur an unnecessary dose of radiation.
      6. No external aiming device to assist with determining the correct angulation.
      7. Potential patient objection to placing the fingers in the mouth.
      8. Potential to be viewed by the patient as unprofessional and unsanitary.
   B. Film holders
      1. Used to position the film packet intraorally
      2. May be used to position the film packet for bitewing and periapical radiographs and for use with the paralleling or bisecting techniques.
      3. Film holder designs range from simple biteblocks to complex instruments that aid in determining the correct alignment of the x-ray beam.
      4. Manufacturers usually offer a set of instruments that can be utilized to expose all intraoral films in all areas of the oral cavity.

II. Bitewing film holders
   A. Designed to hold the film packet in position to image the crowns of both the maxillary and the mandibular teeth.
   B. The placement of bitewing radiographs make bitewing holders unique and different than holders used to position periapical films.
   C. Examples of bitewing holders
      1. Stick-on bite tabs; may be preattached by the manufacturer (Figure 5.6 ■)
      2. Bite loops (Figure 5.6)

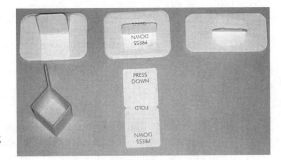

Figure 5.6 Bitewing tabs. Bite loop (left); stick-on tab (center); bitetab preattached by the manufacturer (right).

III. Periapical film holders—paralleling instruments
   A. Requirements
      1. "L"-shaped film holder to provide a stable back for the film packet to prevent bending while maintaining parallel film-to-tooth relationship
      2. Long bite block area to allow for parallel placement of the film packet to the long axis of the tooth (Figure 5.7 ■)
         a. Facial tilt of maxillary teeth requires placing the film an increased distance from the teeth to achieve a parallel relationship between the film plane and the long axes of the teeth (Figure 5.8 ■).
         b. Facial tilt of mandibular anterior teeth requires placing the film an increased distance from the teeth to achieve a parallel relationship between the film plane and the long axes of the teeth (Figure 5.9 ■).
         c. Mandibular posterior teeth are very nearly parallel to the midsagittal plane, and therefore do not usually need a long bite block extension to achieve parallel relationship between the film plane and the long axes of the teeth. (Figure 5.10 ■)
      3. Long 12″ (30 cm) or 16″ (41 cm) PID is required to compensate for distortion that may occur when using a film holder with an increased film-to-tooth distance. (Figures 5.11 ■ and 5.12 ■)
   B. Examples of periapical film holders used with the paralleling technique
      1. XCP film holder stands for *Extension Cone Paralleling*, available through Dentsply Rinn Corporation at www.rinncorp .com (Figure 5.2)

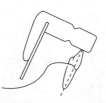

Figure 5.7 "L"-shaped film holder with an extended bite block area for use with the paralleling technique. (Reprinted courtesy of Dentsply Rinn Corporation.)

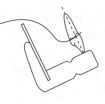

Figure 5.8 Parallel placement of the film packet for the maxilla. Note that the teeth should occlude on the bite block extension to achieve parallel relationship between the film plane and the long axes of the teeth.

Figure 5.9 Parallel placement of the film packet for the mandibular anterior region. Note that the teeth should occlude on the bite block extension to achieve parallel relationship between the film plane and the long axes of the teeth.

Figure 5.10 Parallel placement of the film packet for the mandibular posterior region. Note that the teeth do not need to occlude on the bite block extension to achieve parallel relationship between the film plane and the long axes of the teeth in this region.

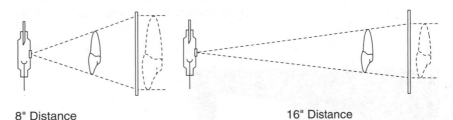

Figure 5.11 Increasing the film-to-tooth distance increases image distortion.

2. Precision-Safe™ film holder available through Masel at www.maselortho.com (Figure 5.4)
3. VIP-2 film holder stands for *Versatile Intraoral Positioner,* available through UPRAD Corporation at www.uprad.com (Figure 5.5)

IV. Periapical film holders—bisecting instruments
   A. Requirements
      1. Ability to retain the film in the patient's mouth; may or may not have a bite block backing.
      2. Bite block backing, if present, is a "V"-shaped slant. (Figure 5.13 ■)
      3. Bite block is short.
      4. Film packet placement is as close as possible to or in contact with the lingual surface of the tooth and is no longer parallel to the long axes of the teeth. (Figure 5.14 ■)
      5. Short 8″ (20.5 cm) or 12″ (30 cm) PID is required to avoid exaggerating distortion, resulting from lack of parallelism between the film plane and the long axes of the teeth.

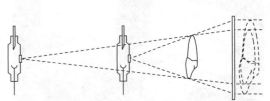

8″ Distance   16″ Distance

Figure 5.12 Increasing the PID length helps to minimize the distortion resulting from increasing the film-to-tooth distance.

Comparing an 8″ distance with a 16″ distance

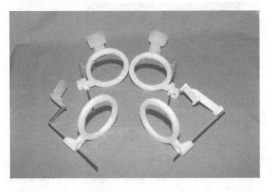

Figure 5.13 BAI (Bisecting Angle Instruments, available from Dentsply Rinn Corporation www.rinncorp.com). Note the "V"-shaped film holder with a short bite block area for use with the bisecting technique.

Radiographic Techniques with Supplemental Film Holders **139**

Figure 5.14 Film packet placement for the bisecting technique. Note that the film should be placed as close to the lingual surface of the teeth as possible.

  B. Examples of periapical film holders used with the bisecting technique
   1. Snap-A-Ray available through Dentsply Rinn Corporation at www.rinncorp.com (Figure 5.3)
   2. BAI film holder stands for *Bisecting Angle Instrument,* available through Dentsply Rinn Corporation at www.rinncorp.com (Figure 5.13)
 V. Periapical film holders that can be used with either the paralleling or the bisecting technique
  A. Requirements
   1. Ability to meet requirements for both techniques
   2. A midlength 12″ (30 cm) PID
  B. Examples of periapical film holders that can be used with both the paralleling and the bisecting techniques
   1. Stabe bite blocks available through Dentsply Rinn Corporation at www.rinncorp.com (Figure 5.15 ■).
   2. SUPA, which stands for *Single Use Positioning Aid,* bite blocks available through Flow X-ray Corporation at www.flowxray.com (Figure 5.16 ■).
   3. Snap-A-Ray, available through Dentsply Rinn Corporation, often achieves a parallel relationship with the mandibular pos-

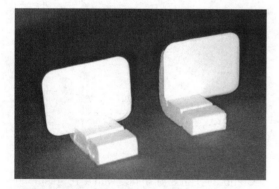

Figure 5.15 Stabe film holder with the film packet placed for a posterior periapical. Note the film packet position in the holder on the right, where the film packet is positioned off-center, allowing it to extend into the posterior region.

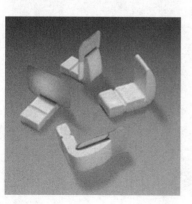

Figure 5.16 SUPA disposable film holders. (Courtesy of Flow X-ray Corporation.)

terior teeth. (Figure 5.3) Also, when held in place appropriately by the patient, parallelism with the anterior teeth is possible.

4. XCP and BAI film-holding devices, available through Dentsply Rinn Corporation, have identical metal extension arms and aiming rings. Switching between XCP and BAI bite blocks allows these instruments to be used with either the paralleling or the bisecting technique (Figure 5.17 ■).

VI. Features of a quality film holder
   A. Simple construction with minimal parts to assemble.
   B. May be labeled or have color-coded parts to aid in correct assembly (Figure 5.5).
   C. Available with instruction manual for learning assembly and use (Figure 5.18 ■).
   D. Easy film packet assembly into and out of the holder without bending. Holder should be able to hold the film securely in place while maneuvering around the oral cavity.
   E. The metal and plastic parts of the instrument should not be imaged, or be minimally visible on the resultant radiograph (Figure 5.19 ■).
   F. The holder should be constructed in such a way to avoid reducing the amount of tissue that can be imaged onto the film (Figures 5.20 ■ and 5.21 ■).
   G. Versatility to image all areas of the oral cavity.
   H. Lightweight construction to enhance the patient's ability to tolerate placement intraorally.
   I. Biting surface made of soft plastic or polystyrene material will provide a secure surface upon which the patient can bite and stabilize the film packet during the procedure.

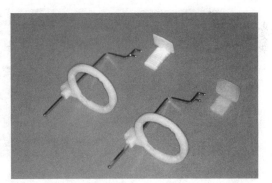

Figure 5.17 XCP film holder on the left and BAI film holder on the right demonstrating identical extension arms and external aiming rings. Note the XCP bite block for use with the paralleling technique on the left and the BAI bite block for use with the bisecting technique on the right.

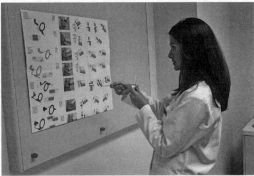

Figure 5.18 Radiographer using the instruction chart to assemble the film holders.

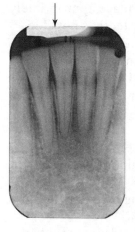

Figure 5.19 Metal prong of the XCP extension arm is often imaged as an artifact on the radiograph.

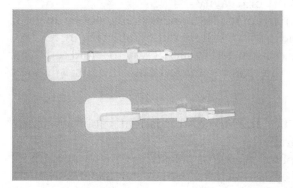

Figure 5.20 Snap-A-Ray film holder demonstrating film packet assembly for vertical (top) and horizontal (bottom) bitewing radiographs. The thick bite block may prevent the patient from closely occluding the teeth, possibly resulting in less image of the alveolar bone ridge.

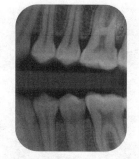

a. Vertical bitewing radio-graph using a film holder with a thick bite block.

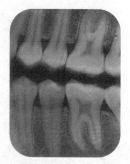

b. Vertical bitewing radio-graph using a thin self-adhesive bitewing tab film holder.

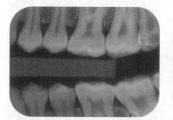

c. Horizontal bitewing radio-graph using a film holder with a thick bite block.

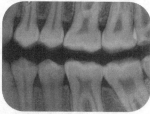

d. Horizontal bitewing radio-graph using a self-adhesive bitewing tab film holder.

Figure 5.21 A comparison of vertical and horizontal bitewing radiographs taken using a film holder with a thick bite block and a self-adhesive bitewing tab.

J. Reusable following sterilization or be disposable.
K. External aiming device (Figures 5.2, 5.4, 5.5, and 5.13).
    1. Assists with determining correct angulation when instrument is assembled correctly.
    2. Aids in aligning the PID over the film packet.
    3. Eliminates the need for precise patient head positioning; for example, films may be exposed when the patient is in a supine position.
    4. Cone-cut error is eliminated when instrument is assembled and used correctly.
    5. Standardization of subsequent radiographs may be easily achieved.
L. External collimator to reduce patient radiation exposure (Figure 5.4).
M. Easily modified to be used with either the paralleling or the bisecting technique. (Figures 4.2 and 5.17)
N. Film holder assembly may be adapted to image special conditions. (Figures 5.15 and 5.22 ■)

VII. Possible limitations of some film holders
A. Multiple instruments required to image different areas of the oral cavity; for example, a separate instrument required for bitewing and periapical radiographs and/or separate instruments for the anterior, posterior, maxillary, or mandibular regions.
B. Multiple instruments required to accommodate different size film packets.
C. Multiple parts requires time and skill for correct assembly.
D. Multiple parts increases the occurrence of incorrect assembly (Figure 5.23 ■).

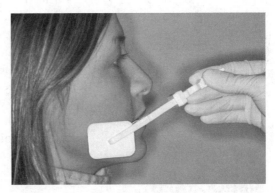

Figure 5.22 Snap-A-Ray film holder demonstrating film packet placement for imaging an impacted mandibular third molar.

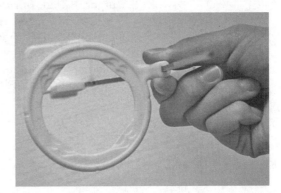

Figure 5.23 XCP film holder assembled incorrectly. Aligning the central x-ray of the x-ray beam to the aiming ring assembled in this manner will result in a cone-cut error.

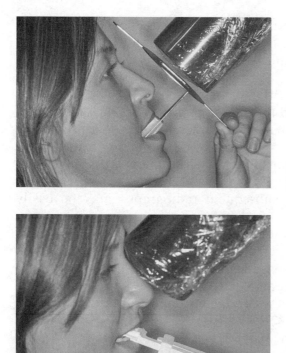

Figure 5.24 The patient may need to hold the Precision-Safe™ film holder in place during the exposure.

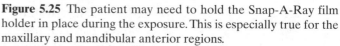

Figure 5.25 The patient may need to hold the Snap-A-Ray film holder in place during the exposure. This is especially true for the maxillary and mandibular anterior regions.

E. Increased time required for assembly of multiple parts.
F. Metal and thick plastic construction may be difficult for the radiographer to place and for the patient to tolerate.
G. Construction of the instrument that results in a reduction of the amount of tissue that can be imaged. (Figures 5.20 and 5.21)
H. Patient may need to assist in holding the instrument in place (Figures 5.24 ■ and 5.25 ■), increasing the chance for movement during the exposure and/or radiation to patient's hands/fingers.
I. No external aiming device to assist with determining correct alignment of the x-ray beam.
J. Infection control protocols required for sterilization of reusable holders.
K. Disposable holders add to infectious waste and have a recurring cost to replace supplies.

BIBLIOGRAPHY

Burger, PA ed. *Intraoral Radiography with Rinn XCP/BAI® Instruments.* Form 1245-289. Elgin, IL: Dentsply Rinn Corporation; 1989.

Dentsply Rinn Corporation: *Green Stabe®.* Booklet #60-0870. Elgin, IL: Dentsply Rinn Corporation; 1987.

Frommer, HH, Stabulas-Savage, JJ. *Radiology for the Dental Professional,* 8th ed. St. Louis, MO: Elsevier Mosby; 2005: 186–215.

1. Which of the following should be used with an 8″ PID?
   - A. XCP
   - B. Snap-A-Ray
   - C. Precision-Safe™
   - D. VIP-2

2. Which of the following provides a means for reducing patient radiation exposure?
   - A. XCP
   - B. Snap-A-Ray
   - C. Precision-Safe™
   - D. VIP-2

3. Which of the following is an *advantage* of the Snap-A-Ray film holder?
   - A. Increased patient comfort
   - B. External aiming device
   - C. Cone-cut error eliminated
   - D. Easy standardization of subsequent films

4. Which of the following might be the *best* choice when exposing radiographs on a child patient?
   - A. Paralleling with Precision-Safe™ film holders
   - B. Paralleling with XCP film holders
   - C. Bisecting with Stabe film holders
   - D. Bisecting with BAI film holders

5. Which of the following might be the *best* choice when exposing radiographs on an adult patient with a large palatine torus?
   - A. Paralleling with Precision-Safe™ film holders
   - B. Paralleling with XCP film holders
   - C. Bisecting with Stabe film holders
   - D. Bisecting with BAI film holders

6. Which of the following is a *disadvantage* of using the patient's finger to hold the radiographic film packet in place?
   - A. Potential film movement
   - B. Potential film bending
   - C. Potential increased radiation exposure
   - D. Potential misalignment of x-ray beam
   - E. All of the above

7. Match the following film holders with the technique *best* utilized with this device:
   - A. Paralleling   _____ XCP
   - B. Bisecting   _____ Snap-A-Ray

   _____ Precision-Safe™

   _____ VIP-2

   _____ BAI

   _____ Stabe with bite extension

   _____ Stabe without bite extension

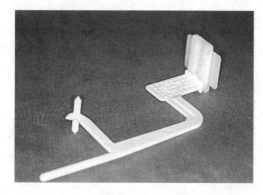

Figure 5.26 Study question 8 refers to this unfamiliar film-holding device.

8. View the unfamiliar film-holding device pictured (Figure 5.26 ■). Which of the following techniques would you expect to utilize when exposing a periapical radiograph with this device?
   A. Paralleling
   B. Bisecting

9. Referring to question 8, what characteristics of this film holder influenced your decision to utilize the technique you chose?

_____

_____

_____

_____

_____

_____

_____

10. It's the first day of your new job. Your patient has been assessed for a full mouth series of radiographs. The film-holding instruments used in this practice are pictured in Figure 5.2. Will you be able to expose all the films you need with the instruments you see here? Identify which of the instrument assemblies pictured will image the (a) bitewings, (b) anterior periapicals, (c) maxillary right posterior periapicals, (d) maxillary left posterior periapicals, (e) mandibular right posterior periapicals, and (f) mandibular left posterior periapicals.

_____

_____

_____

_____

_____

_____

_____

Infection Control and Student Partner Practice

INTRODUCTION

The purpose of infection control is to prevent the transmission of disease between patients and between patients and oral health care providers. Cross-contamination through the creation of aerosols or through invasive procedures is not usually associated with radiographic procedures. However, infectious diseases may still be transmitted through saliva-contaminated radiographic equipment and supplies. Maintaining infection control throughout the radiographic process is particularly challenging. Keeping track of asepsis while moving in and out of the oral cavity can be challenging. Radiographic procedures further complicate the chain of asepsis by requiring movement in and out of the radiographic operatory itself. Furthermore, transporting contaminated film packets to another location, such as the darkroom, for further manipulation can make infection control a daunting responsibility. A thorough understanding of the recommended infection control protocols before, during, and after radiographic services is necessary to protect patients and oral health care providers from the transmission of disease. Additionally, the specific steps of these protocols require practice to achieve competency in skilled handling of contaminated radiographic equipment and supplies.

For this exercise, infection control protocols regarding oral radiography have been divided into four subcategories: 1) infection control prior, 2) during, and 3) after the radiographic procedure, and 4) infection control for the darkroom. While the fourth subcategory focuses on the processing procedure, the first three subcategories concentrate on the operatory where the radiographic procedure will be performed. The purpose of this exercise is to provide the student with an opportunity to practice infection control protocols in these four subcategories. Practice of this laboratory exercise is on a student partner. Through the use of role play, students will simulate exposing a series of bitewing radiographs on each other, establishing a real-life setting in which to practice infection control techniques.

OBJECTIVES

Following completion of this lab activity, you will be able to:

1. Demonstrate infection control protocol prior to, during, and after the radiographic procedure.

2. Demonstrate infection control protocol for the darkroom.

MATERIALS

Student partner

Lead (or lead-equivalent) apron with thyroid collar

Size #2 radiographic film packets

Sterile or disposable bitewing film holder

Patient napkin/bib and chain

Hand washing station with antimicrobial soap or antiseptic hand rub

Disinfectant

Plastic or foil barriers

Paper towels

Disposable cups

Patient treatment gloves

Overgloves

Heavy duty utility gloves

Bitewing film mount

Tomato juice

PREPARATION

1. Study the chapter outline to prepare for this laboratory exercise. An understanding of the material presented in the outline is required to complete this activity.

2. Instructor demonstration may enhance knowledge of the laboratory exercise.

3. Select a student partner. Decide which student will play the role of the patient first and which student will play the role of the radiographer.

LABORATORY EXERCISE ACTIVITIES

Part 1: Exercise in Infection Control Protocol Prior to the Radiographic Procedure

1. Together with a student partner, prepare the radiographic operatory and obtain radiographic materials for this exercise. Follow the infection control guidelines for prior to the radiographic procedure in

Procedure 6.1. Use these guidelines to assess your ability to satisfactorily prepare the operatory for radiographic services.

2. Practice these infection control protocols until all steps can be performed at a mastery level.

Part 2: Exercise in Infection Control Protocol during the Radiographic Procedure

1. Before you begin Part 2 of this exercise, place a small amount, enough to completely coat four size #2 film packets, of tomato juice in the disposable paper cup. The tomato juice will simulate saliva contamination and will be used in part 4 of this exercise.

2. With your student partner playing the role of the patient, proceed with the following steps:

   a. Inform patient of the need for radiographic services, explain procedure and rationale for radiographic services, answer patient concerns/questions regarding radiographic procedure, obtain patient's written consent for radiographic services.

   b. Seat patient.

   c. Request that the patient remove eyeglasses, removable dental appliances, and any other material which may interfere with the radiographic procedure such as chewing gum or facial jewelry adorning the nose, tongue, or lips.

   d. Adjust the height of the chair to a comfortable working level for the radiographer.

   e. Adjust the headrest so that the patient's midsagittal plane is perpendicular to the floor and the maxillary occlusal plane is parallel to the floor when imaging the maxilla and the mandibular occlusal plane is parallel to the floor when imaging the mandible.

   f. Place the lead apron (or a lead-equivalent barrier) with thyroid collar over the patient.

   g. Place a patient napkin/bib over the lead apron. (Figure 6.1 ■)

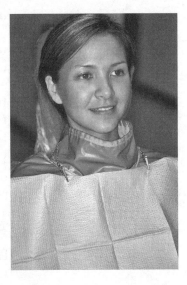

Figure 6.1 A patient napkin/bib may be placed over the lead apron to aid in minimizing contamination of the lead apron.

3. Place each film of the bitewing series intraorally. The size and number of films included in a series of bitewing radiographs for an adult patient is usually four size #2 films. Position the x-ray tube head and PID for each projection. Follow the four basic steps of packet placement, vertical angulation, horizontal angulation, and centering the x-ray beam for exposing bitewing radiographs. (See Laboratory Exercise 2, Bitewing Radiographic Technique.)

   ***WARNING:* DO NOT ACTIVATE THE EXPOSURE BUTTON. DO NOT EXPOSE YOUR STUDENT PARTNER TO RADIATION. YOU ARE PRACTICING FILM PACKET PLACEMENT AND CORRECT X-RAY BEAM ALIGNMENT ONLY. YOU WILL NOT ACTUALLY EXPOSE THESE PRACTICE FILMS.**

4. Follow the infection control guidelines for during to the radiographic procedure in Procedure 6.2. Use these guidelines to assess your ability to satisfactorily prepare the operatory for radiographic services. Practice these infection control protocols until all steps can be performed at a mastery level.

5. Obtain feedback on your packet placement, vertical and horizontal angulation, and centering of the x-ray beam as necessary or as directed by your instructor.

Part 3: Exercise in Infection Control Protocol after the Radiographic Procedure

1. When you have completed taking the simulated bitewing series of radiographs, follow the guidelines for infection control after the radiographic procedure in Procedure 6.3 to secure the radiography operatory.

Part 4: Exercise in Infection Control Protocol in the Darkroom

1. Transport the (simulated) exposed film packets to the darkroom or daylight loader processing area in the paper cup. Ensure that the films are completely coated with the tomato juice. In this exercise, the tomato juice is used to represent saliva contamination. In real life, excess saliva is removed from the film packets by swiping each packet across a disinfectant-soaked paper towel immediately after removal from the oral cavity. (Figure 6.2 ■) While the tomato juice appears unrealistic, it does provide a visible indication of how well infection control protocols are being followed.

2. Process the films following the guidelines for infecton control for the darkroom, Procedure 6.4. If your institution uses an automatic processor equipped with a daylight loader, choose Procedure 6.5.

3. Together with your student partner, use the darkroom assessment tool, Procedure 6.6, to evaluate your ability to follow the infection control protocols.

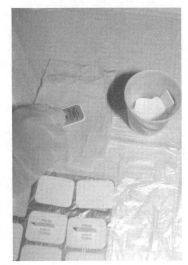

Figure 6.2 After exposure, the film is removed from the oral cavity and immediately swiped across a disinfectant-soaked paper towel to remove excess saliva.

COMPETENCY AND EVALUATION

1. When the exercise is complete, discard films and materials and clean and disinfect the radiography operatory and the darkroom.

2. Switch student partner roles and repeat this exercise. The student "patient" should now play the role of radiographer, and the student radiographer should now play the role of "patient," so that both partners have the opportunity to complete this exercise.

3. Practice these infection control protocols until all steps can be performed at a mastery level.

4. Complete the study questions.

Procedure 6.1

Infection Control Prior to the Radiographic Procedure

Satisfactorily
Performed
✓

1. Put on PPE (personal protection equipment) barrier gown, eyewear, and mask. _____

2. Wash hands with an antimicrobial soap or use an antiseptic hand rub.* _____

3. Put on utility gloves. _____

4. Clean and disinfect with appropriate disinfectant all surfaces that will come in contact either directly or indirectly with the patient. See the following list:

   a. PID _____

   b. X-ray tube head _____

   c. Tube head support arms and handles _____

   d. Exposure button (Push-button exposure switches may be damaged by the use of a disinfectant solution. Maintain infection control through the use of a plastic or foil barrier. [Figure 6.3 ■] Foot pedal exposure switches do not require disinfection.) _____

   e. Control panel dials (impulse timer, kVp, and mA controls) (Control panel dials may be damaged by the use of a disinfectant solution. Maintain infection control through the use of a plastic or foil barrier. [Figure 6.4 ■]) _____

   f. Patient chair including headrest, back support, armrests, body, and back of the chair _____

   g. Lead apron/thyroid collar barrier _____

   h. Countertop and other work space areas _____

5. Wash, dry, and remove utility gloves, and wash hands with an antimicrobial soap or use an antiseptic hand rub. _____

6. Put on clean overgloves. _____

(continued)

Procedure 6.1 *(continued)*

7. Obtain plastic or foil barriers and cover all surfaces that will come in contact either directly or indirectly with the patient. See the following list:

   a. PID (Figure 6.5 ■) _____

   b. X-ray tube head (Figure 6.5) _____

   c. Tube head support arms and handles _____

   d. Exposure button (Figure 6.3) (Foot pedal exposure switches do not require a plastic or foil barrier.) _____

   e. Control panel dials (impulse timer, kVp, and mA controls) (Figure 6.4) _____

   f. Patient chair including headrest, back support, armrests, body, and back of the chair _____

   g. Lead apron/thyroid collar barrier (optional) (Figure 6.6 ■) _____

   h. Countertop and other work space areas (Figure 6.7 ■) _____

   i. Film packets (optional) (Figure 6.8 ■) _____

8. Obtain radiographic supplies. See the following list:

   a. Film packets _____

   b. Sterile or disposable film holders _____

   c. Film mount _____

   d. Disposable paper cup _____

   e. Paper towels _____

   f. Miscellaneous supplies (i.e., cotton rolls, extra disposable film holders) _____

9. Place the film mount under the plastic barrier on the counter work space (Figure 6.7). _____

10. Place the film packets on the plastic barrier placed over the film mount (Figure 6.7). _____

11. Saturate a folded paper towel with disinfectant, and place next to the film mount on top of the plastic barrier (Figures 6.2 and 6.7). _____

12. Prepare antimicrobial mouth rinse for patient use prior to procedure.** _____

* When hands are visibly dirty they must be washed with an antimicrobial soap and water. If hands are not visibly soiled, an alcohol-containing preparation designed for reducing the number of viable microorganisms on the hands may be used. Refer to manufacturer's recommendations for use.

** No scientific evidence indicates that preprocedural mouth rinsing prevents the spread of infections; however, antimicrobial mouth rinses, for example, chlorhexidine gluconate, essential oils, or povidone-iodine, can reduce the number of microorganisms the patient might release in the form of aerosols or spatter during the radiographic procedure.

(continued)

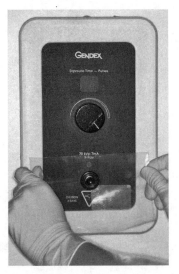

Figure 6.3 Use of a plastic barrier over the exposure button to maintain infection control.

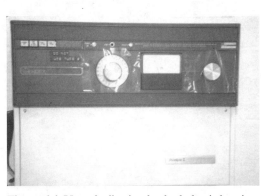

Figure 6.4 Use of adhesive-backed plastic barriers over the control panel dials to maintain infection control.

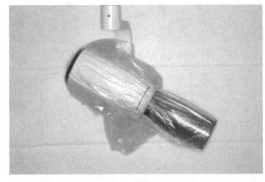

Figure 6.5 Use of plastic bag or plastic wrap over the x-ray tube head to maintain infection control.

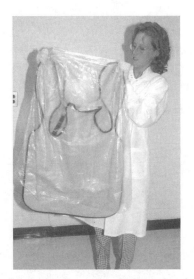

Figure 6.6 A plastic garment bag type barrier may be used to protect the lead apron.

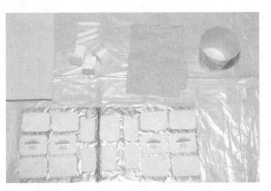

Figure 6.7 Countertop work space covered with plastic barrier and set up for exposure of a full mouth series of radiographs.

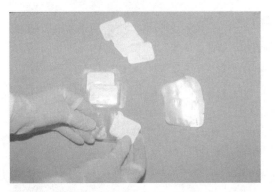

Figure 6.8 Commercially made plastic barrier envelopes may be placed over the film packet to prevent contamination of the film packet.

Procedure 6.2

Infection Control during the Radiographic Procedure

Satisfactorily Performed ✓

1. After placing the lead barrier with thyroid collar on the patient, remove overgloves, wash hands, and put on patient treatment gloves. _____

2. Assemble the film packet into the appropriate film-holding device. Place film packet intraorally and position the x-ray tube head and PID for each of the radiographs in the bitewing series. _____

3. Simulate exposure. _____

   WARNING: **DO NOT EXPOSE YOUR STUDENT PARTNER TO RADIATION. REMEMBER THAT YOU ARE PRACTICING FILM PACKET PLACEMENT AND BEAM ALIGNMENT ONLY AND ARE NOT ACTUALLY EXPOSING THESE RADIOGRAPHS.**

4. Remove the film packet from patient's mouth, following each exposure simulation, and swipe across the disinfectant-saturated paper towel on the counter (Figure 6.2). Drop film into the disposable paper cup receptacle. Do not touch the outside of the cup with contaminated treatment gloves. _____

5. Place and expose all films in this manner. _____

6. If additional supplies are needed that require contact with noncovered surfaces or the procedure must otherwise be interrupted:

   a. Rinse treatment gloves with plain water (no soap) and dry.*

   b. Place overgloves over treatment gloves.

   c. To restart the procedure, remove overgloves.

* If the procedure must be interrupted, the treatment gloves may be removed and discarded and the hands washed. Prior to restarting the procedure, the hands should be washed again and new treatment gloves put on.

Procedure 6.3

Infection Control after the Radiographic Procedure

	Satisfactorily Performed ✓
1. Rinse, remove, and discard treatment gloves and wash hands with antimicrobial soap or use an antiseptic hand rub.	_____
2. Remove lead apron with thyroid collar barrier and dismiss patient.	_____
3. Put on utility gloves.	_____
4. Prepare and package film holders for sterilization according to manufacturer's directions.	_____
5. Discard all disposable contaminated items, that is, disposable film holders, paper towels, cotton rolls.	_____
6. Remove and discard all plastic or foil barriers.	_____
7. Clean and disinfect any uncovered surface.	_____
8. Clean and disinfect lead apron with thyroid collar barrier (if it was not covered with an impervious barrier).	_____
9. Wash, dry, and remove utility gloves.	_____
10. Wash hands with antimicrobial soap or use an antiseptic hand rub.	_____

Procedure 6.4

Infection Control for the Darkroom

Satisfactorily
Performed
✓

1. Obtain two paper towels. _____

2. Place one paper towel on the counter work space, and place the cup with contaminated films on this "contaminated" paper towel (Figure 6.9 ■). _____

3. Place the second paper towel on the counter work space, and keep this paper towel as the "uncontaminated" paper towel (Figure 6.9). _____

4. Secure darkroom door. _____

5. Turn off white overhead light and turn on safe light. _____

6. Put on a pair of clean treatment gloves. _____

7. Open each film packet (Figure 6.10 ■). _____

   a. Peel back the outer plastic/paper wrap using the tab on the back of the packet.

   b. Grasp the black paper with film sandwiched in between and pull straight out.

   c. Hold the black paper-film assembly over the designated uncontaminated paper towel and pull out slowly.

   d. Allow the film to drop out onto the paper towel. Do not touch the film with treatment gloves (Figure 6.10).

8. Drop the contaminated film packet outer plastic/paper wrap, black paper, and lead foil onto the "contaminated" paper towel. _____

9. Repeat steps 7 and 8 until all film packets have been opened (Figure 6.11 ■). _____

10. Rinse, remove, and discard treatment gloves and wash and dry hands. _____

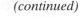

Figure 6.9 Darkroom counter work space with a contaminated area and an uncontaminated area. Note that this setup provides an orderly direction for the progression of darkroom activity. Contaminated film packets begin on the left. Packets are opened, and films are dropped into the uncontaminated area on the right, near the automatic processor loading area.

(continued)

Procedure 6.4 *(continued)*

11. With clean, dry hands, grasp by the edges and place films into the automatic processor feeder slots or load onto manual processing film racks and process following the manual processing procedure. _____

12. When it is safe, turn on the overhead white light, and put on heavy-duty utility gloves. _____

13. Separate lead foil from film packets and discard into lead recycling waste. _____

14. Gather up contaminated paper towel with all waste and discard. _____

15. Clean and disinfect the counter work space. _____

16. Wash, dry, and remove utility gloves. _____

17. Wash and dry hands. _____

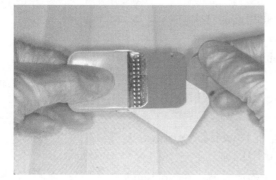

Figure 6.10 Aseptically opening a contaminated film packet.

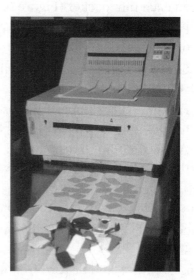

Figure 6.11 Illustration of the contaminated and uncontaminated areas when all film packets have been opened.

Procedure 6.5

Infection Control for Processors with Daylight Loaders

*Satisfactorily
Performed*
✓

1. Obtain paper towels or plastic barrier sheet and new patient treatment gloves. _____

2. Open the light-filter cover, and line the floor of the daylight loader compartment with a clean paper towel or plastic barrier. Designate a contaminated and an uncontaminated side of the floor of the compartment. _____

3. Place the cup with the film packets on the designated contaminated side, and a new pair of patient treatment on the uncontaminated side gloves inside the daylight loader compartment (Figure 6.12 ■). _____

4. Replace the light-filter cover. _____

5. Slide clean dry hands through the light-tight baffles. _____

6. Once inside, put on the pair of clean treatment gloves. _____

7. Open each film packet. _____

   a. Peel back the outer plastic/paper wrap using the tab on the back of the packet.

   b. Grasp the black paper with film sandwiched in between and pull straight out.

   c. Hold the black paper–film assembly over the designated uncontaminated side of the floor of the compartment and pull out slowly.

   d. Allow the film to drop out into the paper towel or plastic barrier. Do not touch the film with contaminated treatment gloves.

8. Drop the contaminated film packet onto the paper towel on the contaminated sided of the floor of the compartment. _____

9. Repeat steps 7 and 8 until all film packets have been opened. _____

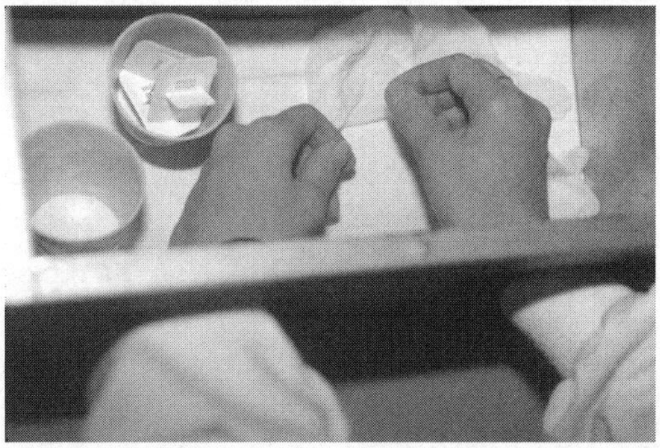

Figure 6.12 Daylight loader work space.

(continued)

Procedure 6.5 (continued)

10. Remove treatment gloves and place on the contaminated side of the paper towel on the floor of the compartment. _____

11. With clean, dry hands, grasp by the edges and place films into the automatic processor feeder slots for processing. _____

12. When the films are safely in the automatic processor, remove ungloved hands through the light-tight baffles. _____

13. Wash and dry hands. _____

14. Put on heavy duty utility gloves. _____

15. Open the light-filter cover, separate the lead foil from the film packets, and dispose of appropriately. Remove the cups, contaminated film packet outer plastic/paper wrap, and paper towels or plastic barrier and discard appropriately. _____

16. Clean and disinfect the inside of the compartment. _____

17. Wash, dry, and remove utility gloves. Disinfect.

18. Wash and dry hands. _____

Procedure 6.6

Darkroom Assessment Tool

Together with your partner, examine the following areas to assess your ability to maintain infection control in the darkroom during the film processing procedure. Place an (X) beside those areas where tomato juice was noted and an (O) beside those areas that remain uncontaminated.

Personal Space

__ Fingers/hands   __ Face/eyeglasses

__ Barrier gown/lab coat   __ Mask

Environment

__ Darkroom door   __ Paper towel dispenser

__ Light switches   __ Outside of processor

__ Walls   __ Outside of lead foil receptacle

__ Counter work space   __ Sink faucets

__ Pen/pencil holder   __Other

I. Goals of infection control
  A. Prevent cross-contamination between patients
  B. Prevent cross-contamination between patient and radiographer
  C. Prevent cross-contamination between radiographer and other oral health care providers
II. Standard precautions
  A. Treat all body fluids (except sweat) as potentially infectious.
  B. Take precautions that prevent contact with all body fluids.
  C. Replaces the term universal precautions where the focus was on bloodborne pathogens.
III. Operator preparation
  A. Use of PPE (personal protective equipment)
    1. Impervious lab coat/barrier gown
    2. Protective eyewear
    3. Mask
    4. Gloves
  B. Handwashing
    1. Remove rings, wristwatches, and other jewelry that can harbor microorganisms.
    2. Lather hands well with soap and rub vigorously for at least 15 seconds, or use an antiseptic hand rub following the manufacturer's directions for use.
IV. Classification of objects used in radiographic procedures
  A. Critical objects
    1. Objects that penetrate soft tissue or bone
    2. No critical objects are used in radiography
    3. Must be sterilized
  B. Semicritical
    1. Objects that contact but do not penetrate mucous membrane
    2. Film holders
    3. Sterilized or disinfected with EPA-registered chemicals classified as high-level disinfectant
  C. Noncritical objects
    1. Objects that do not contact the mucous membrane
    2. Lead apron
    3. Disinfected with EPA registered chemicals classified as intermediate-level disinfectant
  D. Clinical contact (environmental) surfaces
    1. Objects that do not contact the patient, or contact the skin only
    2. Countertops of radiography operatory and darkroom
    3. Disinfected with EPA registered chemicals classified as intermediate- or low-level disinfectant
V. Operatory preparation
  A. Clean and disinfect all surfaces which may be touched during the radiographic procedure.
  B. Spray-wipe-spray technique for most surfaces: spray disinfectant on a paper towel and wipe switches and buttons that may otherwise be damaged by direct spray application.

C. Cover with an impervious barrier all surfaces that can be covered and especially those that are difficult to disinfect.

D. Examples of objects to be cleaned, disinfected, and covered:
   1. PID
   2. X-ray tube head (Figure 6.5)
   3. Tube head support arms and handles
   4. Exposure button (Figure 6.3)
   5. Control panel dials (Figure 6.4)
   6. Treatment chair including headrest, back support, armrests, body, and back of the chair
   7. Lead apron/thyroid collar barrier (Figure 6.6)
   8. Countertop and other work space areas (Figure 6.7)
   9. Film packets (optional) (Figure 6.8)

E. Supplies
   1. Use sterilized or disposable film holders.
   2. Dispense film packets from a central location.
      a. Obtain all film packets required for the procedure at the same time.
      b. Use a clean disposable paper cup as the holding receptacle for transporting the film packets.
      c. Film packets may be prepackaged for ease in dispensing (Figure 6.13 ■).
   3. Plastic film barrier envelopes aid infection control
      a. Protects the film packet from fluids in the oral cavity
      b. The barrier should be opened immediately upon removing the film packet from the patient's oral cavity.
         1) Hold the film packet over the cup designated and open the film packet (Figure 6.14 ■), allowing the sealed film packet to drop into the cup untouched by gloved hands.
         2) Once all of the films are exposed and opened in this manner, the cup will contain uncontaminated film packets that are ready to be transported to the darkroom for processing.
         3) Once the film packet is aseptically removed from the barrier envelope, it may be handled with clean dry hands.

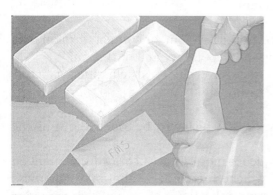

Figure 6.13 Film packets may be prepackaged for ease in dispensing.

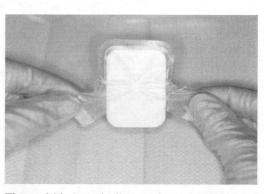

Figure 6.14 Aseptically opening a contaminated film packet sealed in a plastic barrier envelope.

F. Preparation of counter work space
1. Place film packets to be exposed on a film mount that has been covered with a plastic barrier for ease in keeping track of exposures (Figure 6.7).
2. Use a prepared disinfectant-soaked paper towel for removing excess saliva from the film packets (Figure 6.2).
3. Keep overgloves near the counter work space for easy placement over treatment gloves should the radiographic procedure be interrupted.
4. Plan ahead; place extra disposable film holders, paper towels, cotton rolls or other supplies out on the counter work space for easy access.

VI. Infection control during the radiographic procedure
A. Minimize area of contamination.
1. Keep film packets and holders confined to the prepared counter work space area when not in use.
2. Remove excess saliva from film packets immediately upon removing from the oral cavity.
3. Minimize accidental saliva contamination of the lead apron through the use of a plastic barrier or patient napkin/bib (Figures 6.1 and 6.6).
B. Use overgloves if the radiographic procedure is interrupted.
1. To attend to a matter outside of the immediate area
2. To retrieve additional supplies during the procedure
3. To touch an area not covered with a barrier

VII. Infection control after the radiographic procedure
A. Operatory and supplies
1. Use heavy duty utility gloves for cleaning and disinfecting.
2. Remove and discard all barriers.
3. Clean and disinfect all surfaces that were not covered during the radiographic procedure.
4. Prepare, package, and sterilize film-holding devices according to manufacturer's recommendations.
5. Discard all disposable film-holding devices and other materials.
B. Transport exposed film packets to the area for processing
1. Carry disposable paper cup receptacle with exposed film packets to the darkroom or location of the daylight loader processing unit.
2. Handle the disposable cup receptacle by the uncontaminated outside only.
3. The film packet plastic barrier envelopes should be opened, and the films removed in the operatory.
a. Dispose of the contaminated barriers when cleaning operatory.
b. The film packets were protected from contamination in the oral cavity and may be transported to the darkroom for processing.

VIII. Infection control during the processing procedure
A. Darkroom preparation
1. Minimize area of contamination.
a. Designate and prepare an area for contaminated materials.

  b. Assemble necessary supplies, that is, paper towels, cups, pen/pencil prior to opening the film packets.
 2. Clean and disinfect all surfaces that may be touched during the radiographic procedure.
  a. Countertop work space area
  b. Outside cabinet of the automatic processing unit
  c. Sink and faucets
  d. Overhead white light and safelight switches
  e. Pens/pencils
B. Procedure
 1. With treatment gloves on, pull up on the tab on the back of the film packet.
 2. Peel back the outer plastic/paper wrap.
 3. Grasp the black interleaf paper and pull straight out.
 4. Allow the film to drop onto a paper towel (Figure 6.10).
 5. Repeat until all film packets have been opened (Figure 6.11).
 6. Remove treatment gloves and wash and dry hands.
 7. Load the films into the automatic processor or onto manual processing racks with clean, dry hands.
 8. Put on utility gloves.
 9. Discard contaminated materials appropriately.
 10. Clean and disinfect the area.
 11. Retrieve processed films with clean, dry hands.

BIBLIOGRAPHY

Johnson, ON, Thomson, EM. *Essentials of Dental Radiography for Dental Assistants and Hygienists,* 8th ed. Upper Saddle River, NJ: Prentice Hall; 2007: 103–118 .

Kohn, WG, Harte, JA, Malvitz, DM, Collins, AS, Cleveland, JL, Eklund, KJ. Guidelines for infection control in dental health care settings—2003. *JADA.* 2004; 135:33–47.

U.S. Department of Health and Human Services for Disease Control and Prevention, Centers for Disease Control and Prevention. *Guidelines for Infection Control in Dental Health-Care Settings. MMWR* 52(RR17). December 19, 2003; 1–61.

U.S. Department of Health and Human Services for Disease Control and Prevention, Centers for Disease Control and Prevention. *Guideline for Hand Hygiene in Health Care Settings. Recommendations of the Healthcare Infection Control Practices Advisory Committee and the HICPAC/SHEA/APIC/IDSA Hand Hygiene Task Force. MMWR* 51(RR16). October 25, 2002; 1–44.

Wilkins, EM. *Clinical Practice of the Dental Hygienist,* 9th ed. Philadelphia, PA: Lippincott Williams & Wilkins; 2005: 17–21, 52–61, 165–166.

1. All of the following are examples of PPE (personal protective equipment) *except* one. Which one is this *exception?*
    A. Thyroid collar
    B. Protective eyewear
    C. Mask
    D. Gloves

2. Which of these is classified as a semicritical object?
    A. Tube head support arm
    B. Film holder
    C. Lead apron
    D. Treatment chair

3. All of the following must be disinfected prior to radiographic procedures *except* one. Which one is this *exception?*
    A. X-ray unit tube head
    B. Control panel
    C. Film mount
    D. Counter work space

4. All of the following should be covered with an impervious barrier prior to radiographic procedures *except* one. Which one is this *exception?*
    A. PID
    B. Exposure switch
    C. Treatment chair
    D. Film-holding device

5. Which of the following would be indicated for the operator during the radiographic procedure?
    A. Barrier gown, patient treatment gloves
    B. Barrier gown, patient treatment gloves, glasses
    C. Barrier gown, patient treatment gloves, mask
    D. Barrier gown, patient treatment gloves, glasses, mask

6. Which of the following describes the purpose of wiping the film packet with a disinfectant-soaked paper towel following exposure?
    A. To keep film packet moist until processed
    B. To remove excess saliva from film packet
    C. To eliminate the need for gloves when opening film packet for processing
    D. To sterilize the film packet

7. Following exposure, film packets should be transported to the darkroom in a (an)
    A. Coin envelope
    B. Paper cup
    C. Paper towel
    D. Autoclave bag

8. Which of the following should be used when opening film packets *without* plastic barrier envelopes?
   A. Treatment gloves
   B. Overgloves
   C. Heavy duty utility gloves
   D. Clean, dry hands

9. Once films have been separated from the contaminated outer plastic/paper wrap, black paper, and lead foil, films should be loaded into the processor with
   A. Treatment gloves
   B. Overgloves
   C. Heavy duty utility gloves
   D. Clean, dry hands

10. While attempting to place an intraoral film packet in your patient's mouth, you accidentally drop the film packet on the floor. In the space below, indicate how you would maintain infection control in this situation. List specific steps you'd take in responding to this dilemma.

_____

_____

_____

_____

_____

_____

_____

_____

_____

_____

_____

Patient Management and Student Partner Practice

INTRODUCTION

Ideal film packet placement may not be easily achieved on all patients. In radiography, as in other areas of oral health care, each patient presents a unique situation. Although it is important to understand and become proficient in the theory and basic skills required to perform radiographic procedures, the radiographer must be prepared to modify basic techniques. Equally important, the radiographer must be aware of acceptable deviations from the basic techniques which do not compromise radiographic quality. What sets an outstanding radiographer apart is her/his ability to obtain quality radiographic images when adverse conditions exist. Predictable problems with ideal film packet placement have been well documented. Suggestions for overcoming these obstacles should be part of the radiographer's repertoire.

The purpose of this laboratory exercise is twofold. First, this exercise bridges the gap between practice of radiographic techniques on teaching manikins or skulls and performing radiographic services for actual patients. Practice of this exercise on student partners aids in transferring learned techniques from a laboratory situation to clinical application. Second, through the use of role-play, student partners can provide critical feedback not only to improve radiographic technique skills, but also patient management skills.

OBJECTIVES

Following completion of this lab activity, you will be able to:

1. Demonstrate proficiency in placing film packets intraorally and aligning the vertical and horizontal angulation and centering the x-ray beam over the film packet.

2. Maintain an organized and orderly work space area that is conducive to a systematic flow of the radiographic procedure.

3. Determine when to utilize the bisecting technique.

4. Adapt basic radiographic techniques to obtain quality diagnostic images when presented with:
   a. An apprehensive patient
   b. A patient with a hypersensitive gag reflex
   c. Large palatal/mandibular tori/shallow palate
   d. A tight lingual frenulum/large muscular tongue

5. Knowledgeably and confidently respond to patient questions and concerns regarding the radiographic procedure.

MATERIALS

Size #1 and size #2 radiographic films

Sterile or disposable bitewing and periapical film holders

Student partner

Lead apron (or lead equivalent) barrier with thyroid collar

Patient napkin/bib and chain

Hand washing station with antimicrobial soap or antiseptic hand rub

Disinfectant

Plastic or foil barriers

Paper towels

Disposable cups

Patient treatment gloves

Disposable overgloves

Heavy duty utility gloves

Full mouth series film mount

PREPARATION

1. Study the chapter outline to prepare for this laboratory exercise. An understanding of the material presented in the outline is required to complete this activity.

2. Instructor demonstration may enhance knowledge of the laboratory exercise.

3. Select a student partner. Decide which student will play the role of the patient first and which student will play the role of the radiographer.

4. Then switch student partner roles and repeat this exercise so that both partners have the opportunity to complete this exercise as the radiographer and as the patient.

LABORATORY EXERCISE ACTIVITIES

Part 1: Exercise in the Radiographic Procedure

1. Together with a student partner, prepare the radiographic operatory and obtain radiographic materials for this exercise. Follow infection control guidelines for setting up the operatory. (See Laboratory Exercise 6, Infection Control and Student Partner Practice, Procedure 6.1.)

2. With your student partner playing the role of the patient, proceed with the following steps:

   a. Inform patient of the need for radiographic services, explain procedure and rationale for radiographic services, answer concerns/questions regarding radiographic procedure, obtain patient's written consent for radiographic services.

   b. Seat the patient.

   c. Request that the patient remove eyeglasses, removable dental appliances, and any other material that may interfere with the radiographic procedure, such as chewing gum or facial jewelry adorning the nose, tongue, or lip.

   d. Adjust the height of the chair to a comfortable working level for the operator.

   e. Adjust headrest so that the patient's midsagittal plane is perpendicular to the floor and maxillary occlusal plane is parallel to the floor when imaging the maxilla and the mandibular occlusal plane is parallel to the floor when imaging the mandible.

   f. Place the lead apron (or lead equivalent barrier) with thyroid collar over the patient.

   g. Place a patient napkin/bib over the lead apron.

3. Refer to the guidelines for infection control during the radiographic procedure outlined in Procedure 6.2. (See Laboratory Exercise 6, Infection Control and Student Partner Practice.) Place each film of the full mouth series intraorally. The size and/or number of films included in a full mouth series of perapical radiographs varies among practices. Refer to the simulated film mounts pictured in Figure 3.2 (see Laboratory Exercise 3, Periapical Radiographs—Paralleling Technique) to determine the number and size of films that your practice uses. This exercise will use the full mouth series configuration shown in Figure 3.2A. Position the x-ray tube head and PID for each projection. If you are practicing the paralleling technique, make sure that you direct the vertical angulation perpendicular to the film packet plane and the long axis of the tooth. If you are practicing the bisecting technique, make sure that you direct the vertical angulation perpendicular to the imaginary bisector between the film packet plane and the long axis of the tooth. Follow the basic four steps of packet placement, vertical angulation, horizontal angulation, and centering the x-ray beam.

   WARNING: DO NOT ACTIVATE THE EXPOSURE BUTTON. DO NOT EXPOSE YOUR STUDENT PARTNER TO RADIATION. YOU ARE PRACTICING FILM PACKET PLACEMENT

AND CORRECT X-RAY BEAM ALIGNMENT ONLY. YOU WILL NOT ACTUALLY EXPOSE THESE PRACTICE FILMS.

4. When you have placed the film packet correctly and have aligned the x-ray tube head and PID appropriately, have your instructor evaluate your performance and record your progress, using the **Instructor Evaluation and Feedback Form** that follows. Do not wait after each film packet placement for your instructor to initial each projection; instead continue practicing film packet placement, vertical and horizontal angulation, and centering of the x-ray beam. Obtain feedback as necessary or as directed by your instructor.

Part 2: Role-play in Special Patient Management

1. While your student partner is performing in the role of radiographer and working through Part 1 of this exercise, you will assume each one of the following patient roles:

    a. An apprehensive patient
    b. A patient with a hypersensitive gag reflex
    c. A patient with large palatal and/or mandibular tori and/or shallow palate
    d. A patient with a tight lingual frenulum and/or large muscular tongue

    The questions and comments that accompany each of the roles will guide you in acting realistically to challenge your partner to adapt basic radiographic techniques to achieve the goal of producing diagnostic quality radiographs.

2. Throughout the role-play, provide feedback for your partner, both on procedures done well and on those areas in need of improvement.

COMPETENCY AND EVALUATION

1. When the exercise is complete, discard films and materials. The practice films were not actually exposed and will not be processed.

2. Follow infection control guidelines for after the radiographic procedure outlined in Procedure 6.3. (See Laboratory Exercise 6, Infection Control and Student Partner Practice.)

3. When both you and your partner have completed the exercise, each of you should reflect on the experience of being the patient and write out your answers to the following questions.

What strengths did your partner demonstrate as the radiographer?

Why do you consider these strengths?

What specific actions would you suggest for improvement?

How was your partner's "chairside manner"?

What did he/she say to put you at ease with the procedure?

What could have been done better?

Were your questions/concerns regarding the procedure appropriately addressed?

What did your partner say or do to encourage your cooperation with the procedure?

Did you notice other actions during the procedure such as infection control, handling of equipment, attire of your partner, and so on?

What were your thoughts while you were the patient?

Can you imagine your future patients having these same thoughts?

Will they be positive? If not, what can you do to help increase the likelihood of a positive experience for your future patients?

4. Complete the study questions.

NAME _____

INSTRUCTOR EVALUATION AND FEEDBACK FORM

Projection	Instructor's Initials
Right maxillary canine periapical	_____
Maxillary central incisors periapical	_____
Left maxillary canine periapical	_____
Left mandibular canine periapical	_____
Mandibular central incisors periapical	_____
Right mandibular canine periapical	_____
Right maxillary premolar periapical	_____
Right maxillary molar periapical	_____
Right mandibular premolar periapical	_____
Right mandibular molar periapical	_____
Right premolar bitewing	_____
Right molar bitewing	_____
Left maxillary premolar periapical	_____
Left maxillary molar periapical	_____
Left mandibular premolar periapical	_____
Left mandibular molar periapical	_____
Left premolar bitewing	_____
Left molar bitewing	_____

Procedure 7.1

Special Patients Role-Play and Suggested Dialogue

Apprehensive Patient

This patient may be embarrassed by nervous feelings and may not tell you verbally that he/she is apprehensive. Instead, body language, talking rapidly or not at all, and an anxious demeanor may be observed. This patient may have had a past experience with fainting and may fear a recurrence. Nervousness may sometimes prompt the apprehensive patient to assume a defensive attitude and become angry if the procedure is not completed quickly. This may occur as the patient's stress level builds during the procedure. Sample dialogue for role-playing the apprehensive patient:

"Is this going to hurt?"

"How long is this going to take."

"Do you have to take all these films?"

"I don't understand why I have to have this many x-rays."

Hypersensitive Gag Reflex

This patient may talk about gagging prior to the actual procedure or may not bring it up until a posterior film packet is placed. The patient may be embarrassed by this reaction and may get upset that he/she cannot control this urge. This patient may have had an unpleasant experience with gagging in the past, such as vomiting, and may be nervous that it will be repeated now. Or this patient may actually announce proudly that he/she is the biggest gagger you've ever encountered. Sample dialogue for role-playing the patient with a hypersensitive gag reflex:

"I'm a gagger,"

"Last time I had x-rays I gagged."

"Will these x-rays cause me to gag?"

"Can you do something so I won't gag during this procedure?"

Large Palatal or Mandibular Tori/Shallow Palate

Patients with tori do not usually present a problem for radiographic procedures. It is when the torus is large and/or when combined with a shallow palatal vault that placement of the film packet becomes difficult. Large tori prevent alignment of the film packet parallel with the long axis of the tooth and can make it difficult to position the film packet far enough anteriorly to image the canine and first premolar. Mandibular tori may be so large as to extend across the floor of the mouth, making it impossible to place the film into the sublingual area. An additional concern is that the mucosa covering the torus is often sensitive to stimulation. Sample

(continued)

Procedure 7.1 (continued)

dialogue for role-playing the patient with large palatal or mandibular tori or a shallow palate:

"I can't close down."

"Something's hitting the roof of my mouth."

"The film feels like it's cutting the floor of my mouth."

"Can you bend the film or something so that it won't cut?"

"Ouch!"

Tight Lingual Frenulum/Large Muscular Tongue

The patient with a tight lingual frenulum or large muscular tongue may make placement of mandibular periapical and bitewing radiographs difficult. The "tongue-tied" patient may complain of sensitive mucosa as the radiographer scrapes this area in an attempt to place the film parallel to the long axis of the tooth. A muscular tongue that is particularly strong may further interfere with film packet placement by blocking access to the sublingual area. Likewise a tensing of the muscles in the sublingual area may prohibit film packet placement. Sample dialogue for role-playing the patient with a tight lingual frenulum or large muscular tongue:

"My tongue seems to be in the way."

"Where do you want me to position my tongue?"

"It feels like your film holder is too big."

"The film feels like it's cutting the floor of my mouth."

"Can you place the film on top of my tongue?"

I. Special patient management
   A. Be prepared to adapt basic techniques.
   B. Recognize situations that call for adaptation of basic techniques.
   C. Possess a repertoire of acceptable variations of ideal techniques.
   D. Maintain confidence and authority throughout the radiographic procedure.
   E. Be firm yet gentle in instruction to the patient.

II. Apprehensive patient
   A. Causes
      1. Often consider the radiographic procedure to be unpleasant
      2. Unpleasant past experience may contribute to anxiety level
      3. May become apprehensive if the radiographer projects negativity or lack of confidence
   B. Prevention
      1. Develop a rapport that demonstrates attentive listening and empathy
      2. Maintain confidence and authority
      3. Reassure the patient and show appreciation for his/her cooperation with the procedure

III. Patient with a hypersensitive gag reflex
   A. Causes
      1. Psychogenic stimuli—originating in the mind
         a. May be stimulated by the suggestion of a gag reflex
         b. Past experience with a gag reflex may predispose future episodes
      2. Tactile stimuli—resulting from physical touch
         a. Reaction to stimulus blocking the airway
         b. Low tolerance to foreign objects in the oral cavity
   B. Prevention
      1. Maintain confidence and authority throughout the radiographic procedure.
      2. Do not suggest a gagging response if the patient does not bring it up.
      3. If the patient initiates discussion of the gag reflex, allow ample time to communicate concerns; use listening skills to gain the patient's confidence; do not dismiss patient's concerns; empathize.
      4. Explain the radiographic procedure and your prevention techniques to gain the patient's confidence.
      5. Encourage patient's questions regarding the procedure and be prepared to give direct and frank answers to the patient's concerns.
      6. Begin the radiographic procedure by placing those film packets least likely to excite a gag reflex; for most patients this would mean beginning with the anterior film packet placement.
      7. Do not slide the sharp edge of the film packet against the palate or sensitive mandibular lingual mucosa; instead, place directly.
      8. Prepare for the exposure prior to film packet placement, that is, set the exposure factors, estimate the vertical and horizontal angulation, and place and expose the film quickly.

9. Demonstrate placement of the film packet intraorally prior to actual placement by using a finger to massage the tissue.

C. Suppressing once initiated

   1. Begin the procedure over again, utilizing one of the above prevention techniques or the bisecting technique.

   2. Use a distraction technique.

     a. Use a film holder that the patient can be encouraged to clench teeth and bite down on.

     b. Direct concentration to another part of the body during the procedure.

       1) Raise a leg/arm.

       2) Wiggle a finger (Figure 7.1 ■).

       3) Press the back of the head against the headrest.

     c. Employ breathing exercises.

       1) Request that patient hold breath during the exposure.

       2) Request that patient concentrate on taking a number of slow deep breaths during the exposure.

       3) Request that the patient hum throughout the exposure, first explaining that the gag reflex may be initiated by the body's illusion of not being able to breathe.

   3. Individualize treatment.

     a. Before trying any method, whether scientific or gimmick, for suppressing the gag reflex, explain the technique to the patient, allow the power of suggestion of individualized treatment to assist in suppressing the gag reflex.

       1) Use a smaller size film.

       2) Switch to a different film holder.

       3) Apply a cushion to the edge of the film packet (Figure 7.2 ■).

     b. Use stimulation of the senses of taste and feeling to "confuse" the gag reflex.

       1) Request that the patient rinse with an antiseptic mouth rinse or cold water just prior to film packet placement.

       2) Use a film packet that has just been removed from cold refrigerator storage.

       3) Apply a small amount of table salt to the middle or the tip of the tongue just prior to film packet placement.

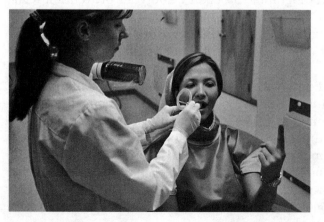

Figure 7.1 Patient attention is directed to another part of the body during the procedure.

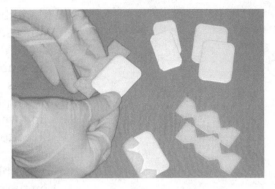

Figure 7.2 Applying a commercially made edge protector to a film packet.

       c. Do not begin the radiographic procedure using any of the above. Instead "save" these techniques to introduce in conjunction with the power of suggestion. (For some patients, especially those who seem proud of the fact that they are the "best gaggers in the world," it may be best to allow for the stimulation of the gag reflex first before trying one of the above methods. Some individuals need to prove that they are gaggers and then will be responsive to suggestions for suppression.)

    D. Severe gag reflex

       1. Apply a topical anesthesia as a last resort.

         a. Introducing a medical agent brings risks.

         b. A numbing sensation, especially in the soft palate and oral pharyngeal area, may cause some patients anxiety and could worsen the gag reflex.

       2. An extra oral radiographic procedure may have to be employed.

IV. Large torus palatinus (maxillary) or torus mandibularis (mandibular) (plural = tori)

    A. Problems encountered during radiographic procedures

       1. Placement of the film packet parallel to the tooth may not be possible.

       2. Film packet may bend during placement.

       3. Patient may not be able to bite down all the way on the film-holding device (Figure 7.3 ■).

       4. Placing the film packet on top of the palatal tori may result in the apices of the maxillary teeth not being imaged onto the film (Figure 7.3).

       5. Mandibular tori may be large enough to extend all the way across the sublingual area prohibiting film packet placement.

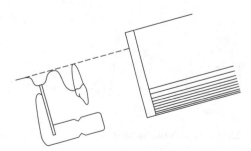

Figure 7.3 Resting the film packet on top of a large palatal torus may prevent the patient from occluding on the bite block of the film-holding device. Note that the apices of the teeth will not be imaged onto the film.

6. Mandibular tori increase the chance of scraping the sensitive mucosa during film packet placement.

7. Large, dense tori appear radiopaque on the resulting image and may obscure diagnostic information.

B. Solutions

1. When placing maxillary periapical radiographs, utilize the midline where the palatal vault is the highest.

2. If the torus is large enough to interfere with film packet placement, place the film packet behind the torus (Figure 7.4 ■).

3. When placing mandibular periapical radiographs, place a finger on the sensitive mucosa over the tori to protect it while placing the film packet intraorally.

4. Apply an edge protector to the film packet (Figure 7.2).

5. When the tori cause film packet placement to be only slightly off from parallel to the long axis of the tooth, a diagnostic image is still achievable by increasing the vertical angulation 5 to 15 degrees (Figure 7.5 ■).

6. When the tori cause film packet placement to be more than 5 to 15 degrees off from parallel to the long axis of the tooth, utilize the bisecting technique, and increase the vertical angulation to compensate for the flat position of the film packet.

7. Large, dense tori require an increase in kVp to allow the x-ray beam to penetrate the structure.

V. Shallow palatal vault

A. Problems encountered during radiographic procedures

1. Placement of the film packet parallel to the tooth may not be possible.

2. Film packet may bend during placement.

3. Patient may not be able to bite down all the way on the film-holding device.

4. If the palate is also narrow, the film may become wedged between the left and right alveolar ridges.

B. Solutions

1. Use a smaller size film with a 5 to 15 degree increase in vertical angulation.

2. Substitute a smaller, lightweight film-holding device.

3. When the palate causes film packet placement to be only slightly off from parallel to the long axis of the tooth, a diagnostic image is still achievable by increasing the vertical angulation 5 to 15 degrees.

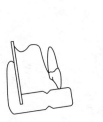

Maxillary film placement

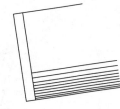

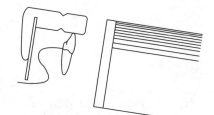

Mandibular film placement

Figure 7.4 The film packet should be placed behind large tori to maintain a parallel relationship between the long axis of the tooth and the film.

186 Laboratory Exercise 7

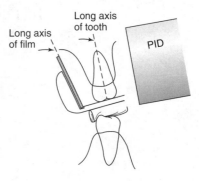

Long axis of tooth

Long axis of film

PID

Figure 7.5 When the lack of parallelism is less than 15 degrees, the resultant image will generally be acceptable. The radiographer may choose to increase the vertical angulation 5 to 15 degrees to compensate for this lack of parallelism.

           4. When the palate causes film packet placement to be more than 5 to 15 degrees off from parallel to the long axis of the tooth, utilize the bisecting technique.

VI. Tight lingual frenulum/large, muscular tongue

    A. Problems encountered during radiographic procedures

        1. Film packet may bend during placement.

        2. Muscular tongue may prevent access to the sublingual area.

        3. Lack of tongue control or an involuntary reaction may prompt the tongue to try to push the film out of the mouth.

        4. If an attempt is made to rest the film packet on top of the tongue, the patient may not be able to bite down all the way on the film-holding device (Figure 7.6 ■).

        5. Placing the film packet on top of the tongue may result in film packet movement and/or the apices of the mandibular teeth not being imaged onto the film (Figure 7.6).

        6. Restrictive tongue movement may increase the chance of scraping the sensitive mucosa during film packet placement.

        7. Tight sublingual musculature may prohibit placement of the film packet parallel to the long axis of the tooth.

    B. Solutions

        1. Massage the sublingual area to help relax the tight sublingual musculature and acclimate the tongue to the position of the film packet.

        2. When placing the film packet, place a finger on the sensitive mucosa over the alveolar ridge to protect it while placing the film packet intraorally.

        3. Before initial placement of the film packet, request that the patient close halfway to relax the tight frenulum and sublingual musculature; as the patient closes the rest of the way, ease the film into place.

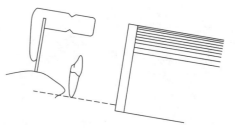

Figure 7.6 Resting the film packet on top of the tongue may prevent the patient from occluding on the bite block of the film-holding device. Note that the apices of the teeth will not be imaged onto the film.

VII. Edentulous areas
   A. Problems encountered during radiographic procedures
      1. Lack of tooth/teeth to stabilize film-holding device.
      2. Film holder may tip into the edentulous space.
      3. No long axis of the tooth to align the film packet parallel to.
      4. Lack of density in the edentulous area may cause an increased radiolucency which may mimic pathosis on the resulting image.
   B. Solutions
      1. Experiment with different film-holding devices.
      2. Use cotton rolls or rolled 2 × 2 gauze squares to "fill" in an edentulous area.
      3. If sufficient alveolar ridge remains intact in the edentulous area, two cotton rolls can be attached to the film-holding device to maintain a parallel relationship between film packet and alveolar ridge (Figure 7.7 ■).
      4. Estimate the long axis of the alveolar ridge to determine the correct vertical angulation.
      5. When a parallel relationship between the long axis of the edentulous ridge and the film packet is not possible, utilize the bisecting technique.
      6. Completely edentulous areas are less dense, and therefore require 25 percent less radiation exposure than those areas with dentition.
VIII. Mal-aligned teeth
   A. Problems encountered during radiographic procedures
      1. Horizontal overlap
      2. Not imaging all the appropriate teeth on one film
   B. Solutions
      1. Increase the number of film packets exposed.
      2. Use two different horizontal angles to overcome overlapping error.
         a. Examine the area of mal-aligned teeth and note the different horizontal angulations needed to complete the image survey (Figure 7.8 ■).
         b. Align the horizontal angulation for the standard exposure, and obtain the first exposure.
         c. Expose a second radiograph, aligning the horizontal angulation such that the x-ray beam will be directed perpendicular through the contact area of the mal-aligned teeth.
         d. When altering the horizontal angulation to expose a mal-aligned area, the film packet should also be altered such that the x-ray beam will intersect it perpendicularly.

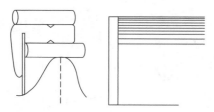

Figure 7.7 If there is sufficient alveolar ridge remaining in an edentulous area, two cotton rolls will aid in placing the film packet parallel to the long axis of the edentulous ridge.

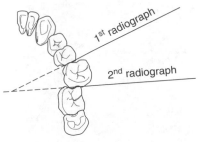

Figure 7.8 Two radiographs, using two different horizontal angulations, may be required to accurately image an area with mal-aligned teeth.

IX. Radiographic procedures for the child patient
    A. Considerations
        1. Smaller oral cavity
        2. Shallow palatal vault
        3. Shallow sublingual area
        4. Fear of unknown procedure
        5. Cooperation levels may vary
        6. Lack of tongue, muscle control
        7. Exfoliating and erupting teeth may lead to increased mucosa sensitivity
    B. Determining the size and number of films to be used depends on:
        1. Oral health care needs
        2. Age of the patient and teeth erupted
        3. Size of the mouth opening and oral cavity
        4. Sensitivity of the oral mucosa
        5. Child's attention span and ability to understand instructions and cooperate with the procedure
    C. Management
        1. Utilize a "show-tell-do" approach to gain the patient's confidence.
        2. Explain the radiographic procedure and what is expected of the patient in understandable terms.
        3. Use smaller film packet sizes.
        4. Modify the film-holding device for patient comfort and manageability (Figure 7.9 ■).
        5. When a parallel relationship between the long axis of the tooth and the film packet is not possible, utilize the bisecting technique.

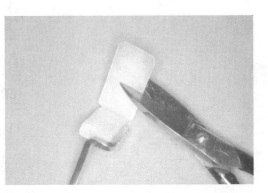

Figure 7.9 Modifying a film-holding device to adapt to a child's smaller oral cavity.

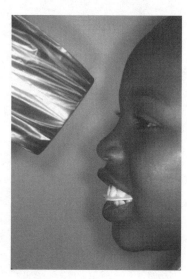

Figure 7.10 Placement of the film packet for use with the occlusal technique is usually well tolerated by the child patient.

6. When film packet placement is difficult, an occlusal technique may be employed (Figure 7.10 ■).
7. When cooperation is difficult, employ caregiver's assistance. Provide the caregiver with the appropriate lead barriers if he/she will be in the path of the primary beam during exposure.

D. Exposure settings for children
1. Children under age 10—Reduce exposure settings to half those used for exposure of adult radiographs.
2. Children aged 10 to 15—Reduce exposure settings by one-third of those used for exposure of adult radiographs.
3. Children over age 15—Exposure settings are the same as those used for adult radiographs.

E. Recommended film size and number
1. Primary dentition
   a. Prior to the eruption of the first permanent tooth (approximately 3 to 6 years of age)
   b. Bitewing examination—two posterior film size #0 or #1
   c. Full mouth examination—one maxillary and one mandibular occlusal film size #2
2. Transitional (mixed primary and permanent) dentition
   a. Following the eruption of the first permanent tooth and prior to the eruption of the second permanent molars (approximately 7 to 12 years of age)
      1) Bitewing examination—two posterior film size #1 or #2
      2) Full mouth examination—ten periapical radiographs (3 maxillary anterior, 3 mandibular anterior, 1 posterior in all four quadrants) film size #1 or #2
   b. Following the eruption of the second permanent molars (after age 12), utilize the same bitewing and full mouth series of films as used for adult patients
      1) Bitewing examination—four posterior film size #2

2) Full mouth examination—14 periapicals (3 maxillary anterior, 3 mandibular anterior, 2 posterior in all four quadrants), film size #2 for all, or a combination of film size #2 in the posterior regions and film size #1 in the anterior regions

BIBLIOGRAPHY

Dentsply Rinn Corporation. *Intraoral Radiography with Rinn XCP/BAI® Instruments.* Form 1245-289. Elgin, IL, Dentsply Rinn Corporation; 1989.

Frommer, HH, Stabulas-Savage, JJ. *Radiology for the Dental Professional,* 8th ed. St. Louis, MO: Elsevier/Mosby; 2005: 177–186.

Haring, JI, Howerton, LJ. *Dental Radiography. Principles and Techniques,* 3rd ed. St. Louis, MO: Elsevier; 2006: 193, 208–211.

Johnson, ON, Thomson, EM. *Essentials of Dental Radiography for Dental Assistants and Hygienists,* 8th ed. Upper Saddle River, NJ: Prentice Hall; 2007: 325–347.

Miles, DA, VanDis, ML, Jensen, CW, Ferretti, AB. *Radiographic Imaging for the Dental Auxilliaries,* 3rd ed. St. Louis, MO: Elsevier; 1999: 136, 143–145.

Thomson, EM: Dental radiographs for the child client. *Dental Hygienist News.* 1993; 6:19–20, 24.

1. Which of the following projections is *most likely* to initiate a gag reflex?
   - A. Premolar bitewing radiograph
   - B. Molar bitewing radiograph
   - C. Mandibular canine periapical radiograph
   - D. Maxillary molar periapical radiograph

2. Which of the following would be the *best* method for preventing a gag reflex?
   - A. Apply a topical anesthetic.
   - B. Use salt on the tip of the tongue.
   - C. Provide instruction confidently.
   - D. Rinse with an antiseptic mouth rinse.

3. All of the following are considered appropriate distraction techniques to help the patient cope with a hypsersensitive gag reflex during the radiographic procedure *except* one. Which one is this *exception?*
   - A. Request that the patient concentrate on the film being placed intraorally.
   - B. Direct the patient to raise one leg during the radiographic procedure.
   - C. Ask the patient to hold his or her breath while the film is being placed intraorally.
   - D. Ensure that the patient is pressing the back of his or her head against the chair's headrest during the radiographic procedure.

4. When exposing a maxillary periapical radiograph on a patient with a large palatine torus, where should the film packet be placed?
   - A. In front of the torus
   - B. Behind the torus
   - C. On top of the torus
   - D. Touching the torus

5. When exposing a mandibular periapical radiograph on a patient with large mandibular tori, where should the film packet be placed?
   - A. In front of the tori
   - B. Behind the tori
   - C. On top of the tori
   - D. On top of the tongue

6. All of the following are considered appropriate actions to help facilitate placement of a film packet when the patient exhibits a large, tight mandibular frenulum *except* one. Which one is this *exception?*
   - A. Massage the sublingual area
   - B. Shield the alveolar mucosa with a finger
   - C. Rest the film packet on the tongue
   - D. Request that the patient close halfway

7. Which of the following adjustments may be indicated for an edentulous area?
   A. Increase the kVp setting
   B. Decrease the exposure time
   C. Increase the distance between the film and alveolar ridge
   D. Decrease the vertical angulation of the x-ray beam

8. All of the following are reasons to alter radiographic techniques for the child patient *except* one. Which one is this *exception?*
   A. Small oral cavity
   B. Lack of tongue control
   C. Increased oral sensitivity
   D. Poor home care

9. Which of the following adjustments to basic radiographic techniques may be required to appropriately image areas with mal-aligned teeth?
   A. Increase the number of films exposed
   B. Decrease the vertical angulation of the x-ray beam
   C. Increase the mA setting
   D. Decrease the size of the film packet used

10. Reflect on your experience today. Having experienced the radiographic procedure as a patient, what insights have you gathered about the procedure? Did you experience anything today that would prompt you to adjust your management of patients in the future?

_____

_____

_____

_____

_____

_____

_____

_____

_____

Film Mounting and Radiographic Landmarks

INTRODUCTION

Dental radiographs should be correctly mounted according to a standardized method prior to viewing and interpretation. Mounted radiographs minimize misdiagnosis, enhance interpretation, and increase efficiency of the viewing process. Radiographic films should be mounted immediately after processing to help protect films from damage that may result from excessive handling. A working knowledge of normal radiographic anatomy will help the radiographer mount films correctly. Although there are two methods of film mounting, the labial method and the lingual method, the American Dental Association recommends the labial method. Standardization of intraoral film mounting will help avoid misdiagnosis. The dental radiographer should be skilled in utilizing the labial method of film mounting, but must also recognize lingually mounted films and understand the two different orientations.

The purpose of this laboratory exercise is to familiarize the student with normal radiographic anatomy and to provide practice in intraoral film mounting.

OBJECTIVES

Following completion of this lab activity you will be able to:

1. Differentiate between labial and lingual methods of film mounting.
2. Correctly mount a full mouth series of radiographs including bitewings, using the labial method of film mounting.
3. Locate distinct maxillary and mandibular anatomical landmarks on a radiographic image.
4. Distinguish between a radiolucent and a radiopaque landmark on an intraoral radiograph.

MATERIALS

Scissors

Film mounts

Sample pre-exposed full mouth series

Viewbox

Highlighter pens (six different colors)

PREPARATION

1. Study the chapter outline to prepare for this laboratory exercise. An understanding of the material presented in the outline is required to complete this activity.

2. Your instructor may provide you with samples of patient radiographs in addition to the simulated exercise presented here.

LABORATORY EXERCISE ACTIVITIES

Part 1: Labial Mounting Exercise (FMS Simulation)

1. Cut out the 20 radiographs on p. 191.

2. Assuming that the embossed dot is raised, i.e., convex, arrange the 20 radiographs on the simulated film mount according to the labial method of film mounting.

3. When you are sure that all 20 films are arranged correctly, secure to the simulated film mount with a piece of tape. The use of removable transparent tape will allow you to repeat this exercise or to change the positions of the films as needed.

Part 2: Labial Mounting Exercise (Sample Radiographs)

1. Obtain the sample patient radiographs from your instructor.

2. Obtain the full mouth series film mount from your instructor.

3. Place the sample radiographs on the viewbox, and arrange them on the film mount according to the *labial method* of film mounting.

4. When you are sure that all the radiographs are arranged correctly, secure in the film mount.

Part 3: Anatomic Landmark Identification Exercise

1. When you have completed the mounting exercises, obtain six different colored felt tip highlighter pens.

2. Using a different colored pen for each structure, highlight the following structures on the images of the radiographs you have just mounted on the simulated film mount page.

Maxillary Landmarks

incisive foramen	BLUE
median palatine suture	GREEN
nasal fossa	PINK
maxillary sinus	YELLOW
zygomatic process	PURPLE
maxillary tuberosity	ORANGE

Mandibular Landmarks

lingual foramen	BLUE
genial tubercles	GREEN
inferior border of the mandible	PINK
submandibular fossa	YELLOW
mandibular canal	PURPLE
mental foramen	ORANGE

COMPETENCY AND EVALUATION

1. List the steps you took to complete the mounting exercises. Discuss why the order of these steps is important. List your own generalizations on how you arrived at the correct arrangement of the radiographs.

2. Explain how a working knowledge of normal radiographic landmarks helped you determine the correct mounting of the films in these exercises.

3. Place the mounted radiographs on the viewbox and role-play patient education with a student partner. The student playing the role of the patient should ask you questions regarding the images viewed on the radiographs. For example, the "patient" may point to the large radiolucent area near the maxillary posterior teeth roots and question the appearance of this region. The student playing the role of radiographer should be able to explain this normal radiographic appearance of the maxillary sinus. Point out to the patient the appearance of the sinus on both the left and right sides. Continue role-playing and quiz your partner on the images you see.

4. Complete the study questions.

Part 1: Simulated Radiographs for Labial Mounting Exercise

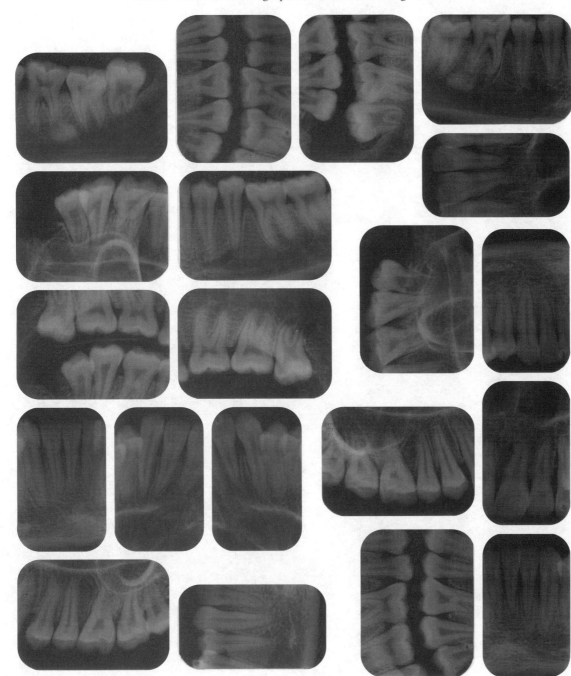

Part 1: Simulated Film Mount for Labial Mounting Exercise

patient's right

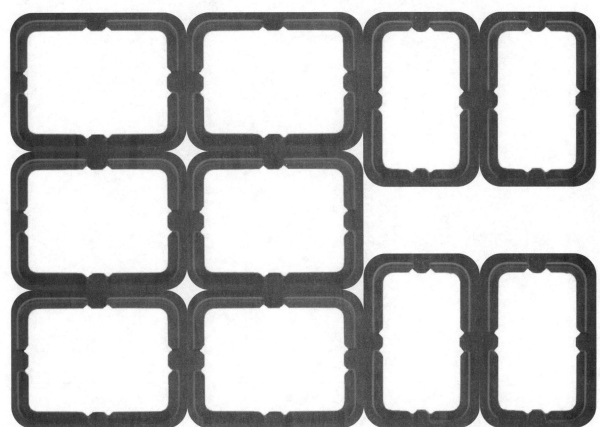

NAME _____

patient's left

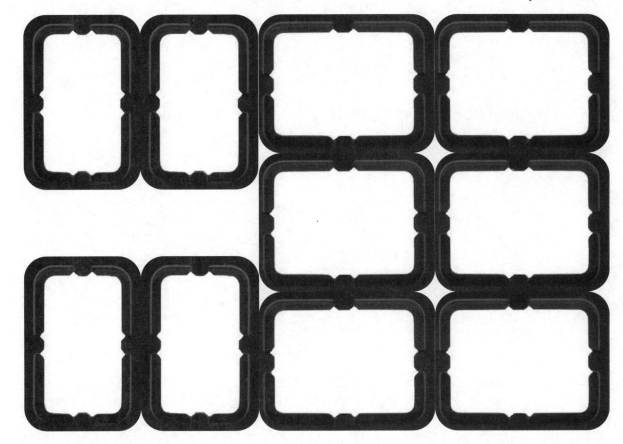

Film Mounting and Radiographic Landmarks   **203**

I. Film mounting
  A. Advantages
    1. Minimizes misdiagnosis by orienting the film in its correct anatomical position.
    2. Minimizes confusing the patient's left and right sides.
    3. Efficiency is maximized when films are viewed side by side, allowing easy comparison between radiographs.
    4. Enhances viewing conditions by masking extraneous light.
    5. Reduces the chance for film damage from excessive handling.
    6. Provides a means for documenting patient information, i.e., name, date radiographs were taken, name of radiographer, facility or practice owner's name.
    7. Aids in charting and documentation of radiographic findings, especially when mounted films and chart diagram represent how the teeth are arranged in the oral cavity.
    8. Aids in patient oral health education and treatment consultations by helping the patient visualize the oral cavity.
  B. Types of film mounts (Figure 8.1 ■)
    1. May be made of translucent or opaque plastic or vinyl, black or gray cardboard.
    2. Window sizes and configurations and number may vary and can be customized to fit the practice needs.
  C. Film mounting methods
    1. Labial mounting method
      a. Recommended by the American Dental Association to establish a standard.
      b. Easily compared with most dental charts, making the transfer of radiographic interpretative findings to patient record easy.
      c. Orientation is "from the lips," as though the radiographer is looking at the patient from a position in front (Figure 8.2 ■).
      d. When viewing the films, the patient's right is on the radiographer's left and the patient's left is on the radiographer's right.
      e. The embossed dot is raised or convex.
    2. Lingual mounting method
      a. Though still used by some practitioners, the American Dental Association recommends the use of the labial mounting method to establish a standard.

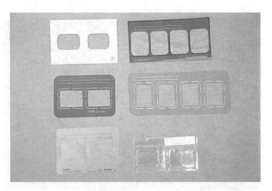

Figure 8.1 There is a variety of film mounts currently available.

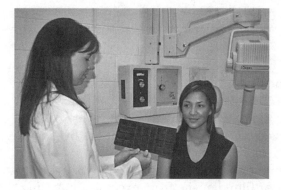

Figure 8.2 With the labial film mounting method, the orientation when viewing radiographs is "from the patient's lips."

    b. Orientation is "from the tongue," as though the radiographer is looking out from a position inside the oral cavity or from a position behind the patient (Figure 8.3 ■).

    c. When viewing the films, the patient's right is on the radiographer's right, and the patient's left is on the radiographer's left.

    d. The embossed dot is depressed or concave.

D. Mounting procedure (Figure 8.4 ■)

    1. Mount films immediately after processing.

    2. Use clean, dry hands.

    3. Handle films by the edges only.

    4. Place films on a light colored counter work space near a view box; use a piece of white paper or light colored tray cover if countertop is dark.

    5. Label and date the film mount and place on the viewbox.

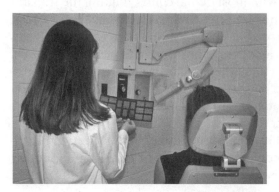

Figure 8.3 With the lingual film mounting method, the orientation when viewing radiographs is "from the patient's tongue."

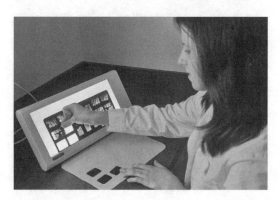

Figure 8.4 Radiographer utilizing a viewbox to mount films.

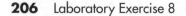

6. Arrange all films so the embossed dots are oriented the same direction, i.e., either all raised (convex) when using the labial method or all depressed (concave) when using the lingual method.
7. Separate films by type of projection, i.e., arrange all bitewing radiographs together and all periapical radiographs together.
8. Arrange periapical radiographs by arch imaged, i.e., place all maxillary films together and all mandibular films together.
9. Orient the maxillary periapical radiographs so that the roots are pointing up, and arrange the mandibular periapical radiographs so that the roots are pointing down.
10. Begin placing the films in the labeled film mount.
    a. Place the anterior periapical radiographs.
    b. Place the posterior periapical radiographs.
    c. Place the bitewing radiographs.

II. Anatomical landmarks
   A. Generalizations that aid in radiographic film mounting
      1. Anterior periapical radiographs (Figure 8.5 ■)
         a. The film packet is oriented with the longer dimension vertical.
         b. Maxillary anterior teeth are generally wider than mandibular anterior teeth.
         c. Maxillary anterior teeth generally have longer roots than mandibular teeth.
         d. Canines generally have the longest roots when compared with adjacent teeth.
      2. Posterior periapical radiographs (Figure 8.6 ■)
         a. The film packet is oriented with the longer dimension horizontal.
         b. Mandibular molar teeth usually have two divergent roots with alveolar bone clearly visible in between whereas maxillary molar teeth have three roots. The superimposition of

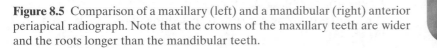

Figure 8.5 Comparison of a maxillary (left) and a mandibular (right) anterior periapical radiograph. Note that the crowns of the maxillary teeth are wider and the roots longer than the mandibular teeth.

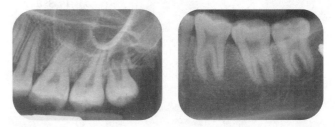

Figure 8.6 Comparison of a maxillary (left) and a mandibular (right) posterior periapical radiograph. Note that the alveolar bone is more clearly visible between the roots of the divergent mandibular teeth, whereas the palatal root of the maxillary molars obscures the view of alveolar bone between the roots.

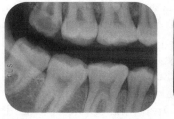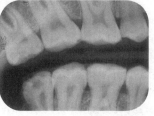

Figure 8.7 When oriented correctly for mounting (film on left), the occlusal plane (Curve of Spee) visible on a bitewing radiograph will appear to curve upward in a "smile" appearance. Note that when the film is oriented incorrectly (upside down), the occlusal plane will appear to curve downward in a "frown" appearance.

the maxillary molar palatal root obscures the view of alveolar bone.

 c. Most roots will appear to curve distally.

3. Bitewing radiographs (Figure 8.7 ■)

 a. Alveolar bone may be more clearly visible between the mandibular molar roots whereas the maxillary palatal root may obscure the view of alveolar bone.

 b. The occlusal plane or Curve of Spee will appear to slant upward toward the distal, giving the bitewing radiograph a "smile" appearance.

B. Identification of landmarks as an aid in radiographic film mounting

 1. Radiopaque landmarks

  a. Dense objects attenuate more of the x-ray beam, leaving less of the beam to strike the film.

  b. Areas appear clear or white to light gray.

  c. Radiopaque areas represent dense landmarks such as

   1) Arch
   2) Bone
   3) Crest
   4) Eminence
   5) Plate
   6) Process
   7) Ridge
   8) Septum
   9) Spine
   10) Torus
   11) Tubercle
   12) Tuberosity

 2. Radiolucent landmarks

  a. Less dense objects allow more of the x-ray beam to penetrate the object and strike the film.

  b. Areas appear black to dark gray.

  c. Radiolucent areas represent less dense landmarks such as

   1) Canal
   2) Cavity
   3) Fossa
   4) Foramen
   5) Fissure
   6) Meatus
   7) Suture
   8) Sinus
   9) Space

C. Landmarks often visible on maxillary anterior radiographs that aid in film mounting (Figures 8.8 ■, 8.9 ■, and 8.10 ■)

   1. Radiopaque

     a. Nasal septum—appears as a vertical, radiopaque bony wall that divides the radiolucent nasal cavity; typically imaged superior to the maxillary central incisors

     b. Anterior nasal spine—appears as a radiopaque triangular-shaped bony protuberance; typically imaged superior to the maxillary central incisors and extending inferior to the nasal septum

     c. Nasal cavity wall—although the nasal cavity is radiolucent, the dense boney wall of this structure appears as a radiopaque outline typically imaged superior to the maxillary central incisors

     d. Inverted "Y"—a radiopaque landmark created by the intersection of the radiopaque outline of the nasal cavity wall and the radiopaque outline of the maxillary sinus wall, typically imaged near the maxillary canine

     e. Soft tissue shadow of the nose—appears as a radiopaque line often imaged as an arc horizontally across the image

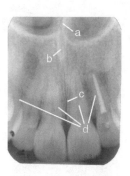

Figure 8.8 a) Nasal septum, b) anterior nasal spine, c) median palatine suture, d) soft tissue shadow of the nose.

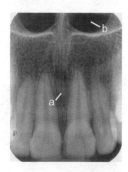

Figure 8.9 a) Incisive foramen, b) nasal cavity.

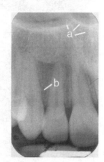

Figure 8.10 a) Inverted "Y" formation, b) lateral fossa.

2. Radiolucent
   a. Median palatine suture—appears as a vertical line beginning between the maxillary central incisors; may mimic a fracture line
   b. Incisive (anterior palantine) foramen—appears as a radiolucent oval between the maxillary central incisors
   c. Nasal fossa (cavity)—appears as paired radiolucent ovals superior to the maxillary central incisor roots
   d. Lateral fossa—appears as a diffuse radiolucency between the roots of the maxillary lateral incisor and canine

D. Landmarks often visible on maxillary posterior radiographs that aid in film mounting (Figures 8.11 ■ and 8.12 ■)
   1. Radiopaque
      a. Zygomatic process (arch) of the maxilla—appears as a radiopaque "U" or "J" shape inferior to or superimposed over the maxillary first molar roots
      b. Zygoma (cheekbone)—appears as a thick radiopaque band extension of the zygomatic process; often superimposed across the maxillary molar roots
      c. Maxillary tuberosity—appears as a raised boney alveolar ridge in the most distal region of the maxilla, yet still remaining on the maxillary bone
      d. Hamulus (hamular process)—appears as a radiopaque spine projecting inferior and distal to the maxillary tuberosity
      e. Lateral pterygoid plate—appears distal to the maxilla; a radiolucent line (suture) may be visible separating the lateral pterygoid plate from the maxilla
   2. Radiolucent
      a. Maxillary sinus—appears as a large radiolucent area extending from the canine to the posterior region of the maxilla, outlined by a dense radiopaque boney wall; appears in almost every radiographic projection of the posterior maxilla
      b. Nutrient canal—appears as a faint radiolucent line extending horizontally across the maxillary sinus on some patients

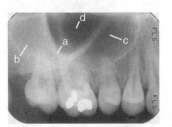

Figure 8.11 a) Zygomatic process, b) zygoma, c) maxillary sinus, d) nutrient canal.

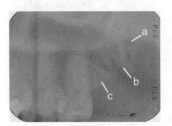

Figure 8.12 a) Lateral pterygoid plate, b) hamular process, c) maxillary tuberosity.

E. Landmarks often visible on mandibular anterior radiographs that aid in film mounting (Figures 8.13 ■, 8.14 ■, and 8.15 ■)

1. Radiopaque

   a. Mental ridge—appears as a sloping radiopaque band inferior to or superimposed over the roots of the mandibular anterior teeth; the two sides of the ridge may actually resemble an inverted "V" when viewed on the mandibular central incisor periapical radiograph

   b. Genial tubercles—radiopaque spines, often appearing in a circle located inferior to the mandibular central incisors

   c. Mandibular tori—appear on some patients as round radiopaque "cotton balls" located inferior to or superimposed over the mandibular teeth

   d. Inferior border of the mandible—if the vertical angulation is increased, the inferior border of the mandible may be recorded on the film as a dense, radiopaque band; the area inferior to this image appears radiolucent or black, representing the space beyond the mandible

   e. Soft tissue shadow of the lip—appears as a horizontal radiopaque line, often visible across the anterior teeth

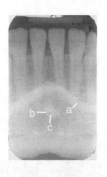

Figure 8.13 a) Mental ridge, b) genial tubercles, c) lingual foramen.

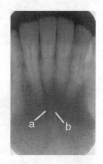

Figure 8.14 a) Nutrient canals, b) mental fossa.

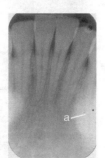

Figure 8.15 a) Mandibular tori.

2. Radiolucent
   a. Lingual foramen—appears as a small radiolucency in the center of the circle formed by the genial tubercles
   b. Mental fossa—appears as a diffuse radiolucency superimposed across the roots of the mandibular anterior teeth; often mimicking a cyst or other apical pathosis
   c. Nutrient canal—appears as a vertical radiolucent line on some patients
F. Landmarks often visible on mandibular posterior radiographs that aid in film mounting (Figures 8.16 ■, 8.17 ■, and 8.18 ■)
   1. Radiopaque
      a. Mylohyoid ridge—appears as a radiopaque line extending from the molar region anteriorly and inferiorly; usually appears inferior to or superimposed over the mandibular molar roots
      b. Oblique ridge—appears as a radiopaque line extending from the ramus anteriorly and inferiorly; usually appears superimposed over the mandibular molar roots
      c. Distinguishing the mylohyoid ridge and the oblique ridge when both landmarks are visible:
         1) The mylohyoid ridge appears more inferior, usually extends further anteriorly, and is not likely to be superimposed over the mandibular molar roots.
         2) The oblique ridge appears more superior and is usually superimposed over the molar teeth.
      d. Inferior border of the mandible—if the vertical angulation is increased, the inferior border of the mandible may be

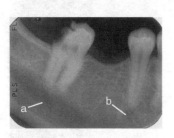

Figure 8.16 a) Oblique ridge, b) mylohyoid ridge, c) inferior border of the mandible.

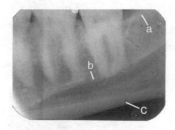

Figure 8.17 a) Submandibular fossa, b) mental foramen.

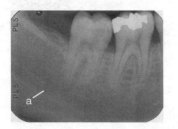

Figure 8.18 a) Mandibular canal.

212 Laboratory Exercise 8

recorded on the film as a dense, radiopaque band; the area inferior to this image appears radiolucent or black, representing the space beyond the mandible

    e. Mandibular tori—appear on some patients as round radiopaque "cotton balls" located inferior to or superimposed over the mandibular teeth

  2. Radiolucent

    a. Mental foramen—appears as a circular radiolucency near the mandibular second premolar root; often mimicking periapical pathosis

    b. Mandibular canal—appears as a radiolucent horizontal canal outlined by parallel radiopaque lines (canal walls) traversing the mandible; the mandibular canal appears inferior to or superimposed over the mandibular posterior teeth roots

    c. Submandibular fossa—appears as a large radiolucency in the posterior body of the mandible inferior to the mylohyoid ridge

    d. Nutrient canal—appears as a vertical radiolucent line on some patients

BIBLIOGRAPHY

Haring, JI, Howerton, LJ. *Dental Radiography. Principles and Techniques,* 3rd ed. St. Louis, MO: Elsevier; 2006: 368–406.

Haring, JI, Lind, LJ. *Radiographic Interpretation for the Dental Hygienist.* Philadelphia, PA: WB Saunders Co; 1993: 25–52.

Film Mounting and Radiographic Landmarks   **213**

1. All of the following are advantages of film mounting *except* one. Which one is this *exception?*
   A. Minimizes misdiagnosis
   B. Reduces the chance for film damage
   C. Eliminates the need for duplicate radiographs
   D. Aids in charting and documentation

2. Which of the following methods of film mounting is recommended by the American Dental Association?
   A. Labial method
   B. Lingual method

3. Which of the following indicates the labial method of film mounting?
   A. Embossed dot is convex, viewer orientation is facing the patient
   B. Embossed dot is concave, viewer orientation is facing the patient
   C. Embossed dot is convex, viewer orientation is facing in the same direction as the patient
   D. Embossed dot is concave, viewer orientation is facing in the same direction as the patient

4. Which of the following is *false* when using generalizations as an aid to film mounting?
   A. Maxillary anterior teeth are wider then mandibular anterior teeth.
   B. Mandibular molars have two roots while maxillary molars have three.
   C. Most roots curve mesially.
   D. The occlusal plane curves upward into a "smile" appearance.

5. Which of the following would appear *radiolucent* on a radiograph?
   A. Maxillary sinus
   B. Anterior nasal spine
   C. Genial tubercles
   D. Mental ridge

6. Which of the following would appear *radiopaque* on a radiograph?
   A. Incisive foramen
   B. Median palatine suture
   C. Mental foramen
   D. Mylohyoid ridge

7. All of the following would be likely to appear on a maxillary anterior radiograph *except* one. Which one is this *exception?*
   A. Maxillary tuberosity
   B. Nasal septum
   C. Incisive foramen
   D. Lateral fossa

8. All of the following would be likely to appear on a maxillary posterior radiograph *except* one. Which one is this *exception?*
   - A. Hamulus
   - B. Nasal fossa
   - C. Zygomatic process
   - D. Lateral pterygoid plate

9. All of the following would be likely to appear on a mandibular anterior radiograph *except* one. Which one is this *exception?*
   - A. Mental foramen
   - B. Genial tubercles
   - C. Lingual foramen
   - D. Mental ridge

10. All of the following would be likely to appear on a mandibular posterior radiograph *except* one. Which one is this *exception?*
    - A. Mental fossa
    - B. Submandibular fossa
    - C. Mandibular canal
    - D. Oblique ridge

Exposure Variables—Factors Affecting the Radiographic Image

INTRODUCTION

Producing diagnostic quality radiographic images is the radiographer's goal. A multitude of factors influences the quality of the radiographic image produced. It is important to understand the role variations in, and relationships between, these factors play in producing a radiographic image. Equally important is the radiographer's ability to tailor the radiation exposure to fit the patient's needs. The x-ray beam can be altered to reduce radiation exposure in edentulous areas, anterior regions, and, for the child patient, while still maintaining consistent image density and contrast. Further alterations in the variables that control image contrast can be made to improve diagnosis of caries versus a periodontal assessment. Being able to accurately adjust the factors that influence radiographic quality can produce diagnostically superior radiographs while minimizing radiation exposure. Because not all factors affecting the radiographic image can be controlled by the radiographer, an understanding of the effect these variables have on the radiographic image will prepare the radiographer to interpret a quality image.

The factors affecting the radiographic image can be divided into four categories. The visual appearance of a radiographic image can be affected by altering (1) beam factors, (2) subject/object factors, (3) film factors, or (4) geometric factors. The effects of these variables are interrelated. While changing one factor can change the visual characteristics of the radiographic image, changing multiple factors, designed to offset each other, may produce similar images.

Beam Factors

The intensity and penetrating ability of the x-ray beam has a major effect on the image density and contrast. The amount of radiation reaching the film is governed by the milliamperage setting, while the strength or quality of the x-ray beam is controlled by the kilovoltage setting. The exposure timer or impulse setting determines the length of time the patient is exposed to the set intensity and strength of the x-ray beam. Traditionally, dental x-ray equipment has been designed to allow the radiographer to adjust the three beam factors of milliamperage, kilovoltage, and exposure time. Technology has made available modern x-ray equipment with preset technique variables, so the radiographer who possesses a working knowledge of the effects and countereffects of changing one variable or multiple variables may be better prepared to evaluate the quality of radiographic images produced by these preset machines. All dental x-ray machines have a variable exposure timer.

Subject/Object Factors

For the purposes of dental radiographic imagery, it is important to note that subject factors such as size of the patient and density of the tooth structure can affect the visual characteristics of the radiographic image. Thicker subjects/objects attenuate more x-ray photons, reducing the amount of x-rays that reach the film. Additionally, denser objects, those with a higher atomic number, will also prevent x-rays from reaching the film. Because subject/object factors are beyond the control of the radiographer, counter adjustments in the other factor categories may be necessary to achieve proper density and contrast of the radiographic image.

Film Factors

Currently film speeds available for use in producing dental radiographs include "D," "E," and "F" speeds. The American Dental Association and the American Academy of Oral and Maxillofacial Radiology recommend the use of the fastest speed film currently available because of its reduction in patient radiation dose. However, some clinicians still prefer to use "D" speed film because of its purported visual clarity. While this reasoning is debated, the dental radiographer should be aware that varying film speeds may affect the visual characteristics of the radiographic image and that appropriate variable counter adjustments must be made when switching film speeds.

Geometric Factors

The PID length, or target-to-film distance, plays a major role in affecting the radiographic image. The length of the PID can be compared with a shadow cast principle. Shadow cast principles are considered geometric variables. The five shadow cast principles are to utilize (1) a small focal spot size; (2) a long target-to-film distance; (3) a short object-to-film distance; and maintain (4) a parallel relationship between the plane of the film packet and the long axis of the tooth; and (5) a perpendicular relationship between the x-ray beam and both the film packet and the long axis of the tooth. If all shadow cast principles are met, then the resultant radiographic image is considered a perfect representation of the anatomical structures being radiographed. However, neither the paralleling nor the bisecting technique can satisfy all shadow cast principles in all regions of the oral cavity. The radiographer's goal is to follow as many shadow cast principles as possible. The first principle is preset by the manufacturer of the x-ray unit and beyond the control of the radiographer. When utilizing the paralleling technique, the radiographer achieves the fourth and fifth principles, but not the third, and the bisecting technique allows the radiographer to meet the third principle, but not the fourth and fifth. The second shadow cast principle, which states that the distance between the target (inside the tube head) and the film should be increased, translates into the recommendation of the use of a long 16-inch or 12-inch PID versus an 8-inch PID (Figure 9.1 ■). The use of a long PID reduces image magnification. (See Figure 5.12.) A long PID is especially necessary when utilizing the paralleling technique. To achieve parallel film packet placement necessary for the paralleling technique, the film is usually placed a greater distance away from the tooth, which contributes to image magnification. A long PID increases the distance between the target and film and helps to compensate for this magnification. Although the use of a long PID is recommended, some radiographers find it difficult to maneuver into place, especially when utilizing the bisecting technique which usually requires increased vertical angulation. Currently a midlength 12-inch PID is available for use with most dental x-ray machines. The 12-inch PID may be less cumbersome than the 16-inch PID and yet still increase the target-to-film distance over the 8-inch PID. Some dental x-ray units have a recessed PID, which provides an increased target-to-film distance by recessing the target into the back of the tube head (Figure 9.2 ■). Some x-ray units allow the

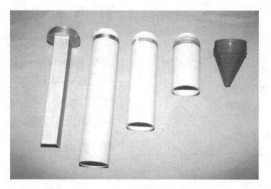

Figure 9.1 PID (position indicating device) lengths and shapes. L-R: 16″ (41 cm) open-ended rectangular; 16″ (41 cm) open-ended circular; 12″ (30 cm) open-ended circular; 8 (20.5 cm) open-ended circular; and 4″ (10 cm) closed-ended pointed (no longer recommended because of the increase in scatter radiation and the increased radiation dose to the patient).

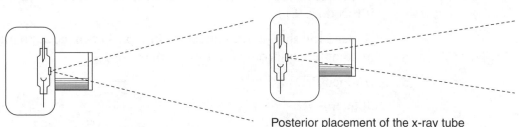

Anterior placement of the x-ray tube in the x-ray unit tube head.

Posterior placement of the x-ray tube in the x-ray unit tube head. (Recessed design)

Figure 9.2 A seemingly short PID may indeed be longer than it appears. Traditionally the vacuum tube, where x-rays originate, has been located in the anterior part of the tube head. A recessed design places the tube in the posterior part of the tube head, thus increasing the distance the x-rays must travel to reach the film.

Exposure Variables—Factors Affecting the Radiographic Image **219**

radiographer to change PID lengths. When altering the length of the PID, a corresponding adjustment to the exposure time must be made to maintain film density. Changing the target-to-film distance requires a working knowledge of the inverse square law.

The dental radiographer should be able to identify situations that may call for an alteration in the radiograph technique settings. A skilled dental radiographer will possess a working knowledge of the factors affecting the radiographic image and make accurate adjustments to produce diagnostic quality radiographs.

The purpose of this laboratory exercise is to demonstrate the effect of varying (1) beam factors, (2) object/subject factors, (3) film factors, and (4) geometric factors on the resultant radiographic image.

OBJECTIVES

Following completion of this lab activity, you will be able to:

1. Identify factors that influence radiographic density.

2. Identify factors that influence radiographic contrast.

3. Appropriately adjust technique settings to increase/decrease radiographic image density/contrast.

4. Appropriately adjust the exposure time when altering the PID length.

MATERIALS

Teaching manikin or skull

Lead (or lead equivalent) apron and thyroid collar

Size #2 radiographic films (one film should be a slower speed; e.g., if using "F" speed film for all exercises, have one "E" or "D" speed film available for use in Part 5)

Periapical film-holding device

Viewbox

1 large paper clip and 1 small paper clip

Step-wedge (commercially made or made from discarded lead foils using Procedure 9.1)

12 lead foil sheets from intraoral film packets needed to make step-wedge if commercial product not available

16-inch PID

8-inch PID

PREPARATION

1. Study the chapter outline to prepare for this laboratory exercise. An understanding of the material presented in the outline is required to complete this activity.

2. Prepare radiology operatory. Set up teaching manikin or skull. Ensure that correct "patient" positioning is achieved, i.e., occlusal plane parallel to the floor, midsagittal plane perpendicular to the floor.

3. Place lead apron (or lead-equivalent barrier) and thyroid collar over the "patient."

4. Instructor demonstration may enhance knowledge of the laboratory exercise.

LABORATORY EXERCISE ACTIVITIES

Part 1: Effect of Exposure Time on Film Density

1. Obtain three size #2 radiographic film packets.

2. Prepare to expose the maxillary central incisor periapical radiograph. Place film packets in the film-holding device.

3. Check posted exposure settings for the dental x-ray unit, and set for the maxillary central incisor periapical radiograph.

4. Place the first film packet and expose the maxillary central incisor periapical radiograph using the paralleling technique.

5. Next, check the posted exposure settings **AND INCREASE THE EXPOSURE TIME BY ONE-HALF.** For example, if your posted exposure settings chart recommends an exposure time of 16 impulses for proper exposure of the maxillary central incisor periapical radiograph, you would now increase that exposure time to 24 (16 + 8 = 24).

6. Place the large paper clip on the second film packet to help you identify this film after processing. Place the second film packet, and expose the maxillary central incisor periapical radiograph using the paralleling technique at this **INCREASED** exposure setting.

7. Next check the posted exposure settings **AND DECREASE THE ORIGINAL EXPOSURE TIME BY ONE-HALF.** For example, if your posted exposure settings chart recommends an exposure time of 16 impulses for proper exposure of the maxillary central incisor periapical radiograph, you would now decrease that exposure time to 8 (16 − 8 = 8).

8. Place the small paper clip on the third film packet to help you identify this film after processing. Place the third film packet and expose the maxillary central incisor periapical radiograph using the paralleling technique at this **DECREASED** exposure setting.

9. Process the three films.

Part 2: Effect of Milliamperage on Film Density

1. Obtain two size #2 radiographic film packets.

2. Prepare to expose the maxillary central incisor periapical radiograph. Place film packets in the film-holding device.

3. Check posted exposure settings for the dental x-ray unit, set for the maxillary central incisor periapical radiograph, **AND SET THE MILLIAMPERAGE AT THE HIGHEST POSSIBLE SETTING.**

4. Place the large paper clip on the first film packet to help you identify this film after processing. Place the first film packet and expose the maxillary central incisor periapical radiograph using the paralleling technique at this **INCREASED** milliamperage setting.

5. Next check the posted exposure settings for the dental x-ray unit, set for the maxillary central incisor periapical radiograph, **AND SET THE MILLIAMPERAGE AT THE LOWEST POSSIBLE SETTING.**

6. Place the small paper clip on the second film packet to help you identify this film after processing. Place the second film packet and expose the maxillary central incisor periapical radiograph using the paralleling technique at this **DECREASED** milliamperage setting.

7. Process the two films.

Part 3: Effect of Kilovoltage Setting on Film Density

1. Obtain two size #2 radiographic film packets.

2. Prepare to expose the maxillary central incisor periapical radiograph. Place film packets in the film-holding device.

3. Check posted exposure settings for the dental x-ray unit, set for the maxillary central incisor periapical radiograph, **AND SET THE KILO-VOLTAGE AT THE HIGHEST POSSIBLE SETTING.**

4. Place the large paper clip on the first film packet to help you identify this film after processing. Place the first film packet and expose the maxillary central incisor periapical radiograph using the paralleling technique at this **INCREASED** kilovoltage setting.

5. Next check the posted exposure settings for the dental x-ray unit, set for the maxillary central incisor periapical radiograph, **AND SET THE KILOVOLTAGE AT THE LOWEST POSSIBLE SETTING.**

6. Place the small paper clip on the second film packet to help you identify this film after processing. Place the second film packet and expose the maxillary central incisor periapical radiograph using the paralleling technique at this **DECREASED** kilovoltage setting.

7. Process the two films.

PART 4: EFFECT OF KILOVOLTAGE SETTING ON FILM CONTRAST

1. Designate an area, countertop or operatory chair, for this exercise.

2. Using Procedure 9.1, prepare a step wedge or use a commercially manufactured device (Figure 9.3 ■).

3. Obtain two size #2 radiographic film packets.

4. Check posted exposure settings for the dental x-ray unit, and set for the maxillary central incisor periapical radiograph.

5. Next **SET THE KILOVOLTAGE AT THE HIGHEST POSSIBLE SETTING.**

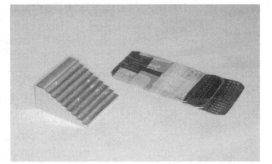

Figure 9.3 A commercially manufactured step wedge on the left and a model assembled from intraoral film packet lead foil sheets on the right.

6. Prepare to expose the first film by placing it tube side up on the countertop or operatory chair.

7. Place the large paper clip on the film to help you identify this film after processing.

8. Place the step wedge on top of the film packet, on top of the paper clip.

9. Direct the PID over the film packet and step wedge. Maintain a distance of 1″ between the edge of the PID and the film packet step wedge (Figure 9.4 ■).

10. Expose the film and step wedge at this **INCREASED** kilovoltage setting.

11. Next check the posted exposure settings for the dental x-ray unit, set for the maxillary central incisor periapical radiograph, **AND SET THE KILOVOLTAGE AT THE LOWEST POSSIBLE SETTING.**

12. Prepare to expose the second film by placing it tube side up on the countertop or operatory chair.

13. Place the small paper clip on the film to help you identify this film after processing.

14. Place the step wedge on top of the film packet.

15. Direct the PID over the film packet and step wedge. Maintain a distance of 1″ between the edge of the PID and the film packet-step wedge (Figure 9.4).

16. Expose the film and step wedge at this **DECREASED** kilovoltage setting.

17. Process the two films.

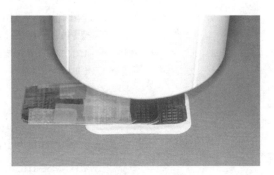

Figure 9.4 Assembled step wedge and film packet ready for exposure. Note that the PID is in position approximately 1 inch above the film.

Exposure Variables—Factors Affecting the Radiographic Image **223**

Part 5: Effect of Film Speed on Film Density

1. Obtain one each of the "F" speed (use the fastest speed film available) and the "D" speed (use the slowest film speed available) size #2 radiographic film packets.

2. Prepare to expose the maxillary central incisor periapical radiograph. Place the "F" speed film packet in the film-holding device.

3. Check posted exposure settings for the dental x-ray unit, and set for the maxillary central incisor periapical radiograph using "F" speed film.

4. Place and expose the maxillary central incisor periapical radiograph using the paralleling technique.

5. Next, **PLACE THE "D" SPEED FILM PACKET** in the film-holding device.

6. Place the small paper clip on the "D" speed film to help you identify this film after processing.

7. **DO NOT CHANGE ANY EXPOSURE SETTINGS.** Instead place and expose the maxillary central incisor periapical radiograph using the paralleling technique with the "D" speed film **USING THE "F" SPEED SETTINGS.**

8. Process the two films.

Part 6: Effect of PID Length on Film Density and the Inverse Square Law

1. Obtain three size #2 radiographic film packets.

2. Prepare to expose the maxillary central incisor periapical radiograph. Place film packets in the film-holding device.

3. Check posted exposure settings for the dental x-ray unit, and set for the maxillary central incisor periapical radiograph and the **16″ PID.**

4. Place the first film packet, and expose the maxillary central incisor periapical radiograph using the paralleling technique and the **16″ PID.**

5. Next, **REMOVE THE 16″ PID AND REPLACE WITH AN 8″ PID. DO NOT CHANGE THE EXPOSURE SETTINGS.**

6. Place the large paper clip on the second film packet to help you identify this film after processing. Place the second film packet and expose the maxillary central incisor periapical radiograph using the paralleling technique at this **DECREASED** PID length.

7. Next take the exposure settings you just used, **AND DECREASE THE IMPULSE TIME BY 4.** For example, if you used an exposure impulse time of 16, you would now decrease that exposure time to 4 ($16 \div 4 = 4$).

8. Place the small paper clip on the third film packet to help you identify this film after processing. Place the third film packet and expose the maxillary central incisor periapical radiograph using the paralleling technique with the 8″ PID at this **DECREASED** exposure setting.

9. Process the three films.

1. Mount the processed films on the simulated film mount pages that follow. Secure with a piece of tape placed along the top edge of the film only, so that the films may be raised slightly, to allow light underneath for ease of viewing. The use of removable transparent tape will allow the film mount page to be used more than once.

    NOTE: Use the labial mounting method. (See Laboratory Exercise 8, Film Mounting and Radiographic Landmarks, for details.) The raised portion of the embossed dot is toward you (convex) when placing the film onto the page.

2. Using the space under each simulated film mount, record the exposure settings you used for each of the six parts of this exercise.

3. Place the page with the mounted films taped to it on a view box and evaluate.

4. Examine the resultant radiographic images in each of the six parts of this exercise. Based on your results, summarize the following in your own words:

    a. What is the effect of altering the exposure time on the radiographic image?

    b. What is the effect of altering the milliamperage on the radiographic image?

    c. What is the effect of altering the kilovoltage on the radiographic image?

    d. What is the effect of altering the film speed on the radiographic image?

    e. What is the effect of altering the PID length on the radiographic image?

    f. How would you compensate for a change in PID length so that the resultant image will stay the same?

NAME _____

Standard exposure
(No paper clip)

Increased exposure time
(Large paper clip)

Decreased exposure time
(Small paper clip)

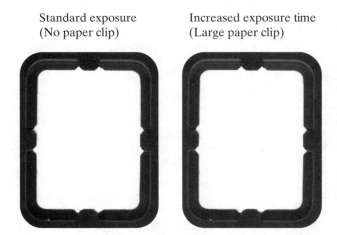

Record the technique settings used for this exercise below.

Standard exposure:
mA _____
kVp _____
impulses _____

Increased exposure time:
mA _____
kVp _____
impulses _____

Decreased exposure time:
mA _____
kVp _____
impulses _____

Part 2: Effect of Milliamperage on Film Density

Increased milliamerage
(Large paper clip)

Decreased milliamperage
(Small paper clip)

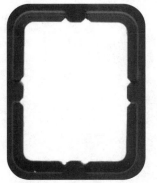
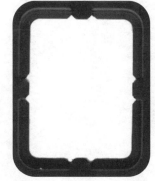

Record the technique settings used for this exercise below.

Increased milliamperage:
mA _____
kVp _____
impulses _____

Decreased milliamperage:
mA _____
kVp _____
impulses _____

Part 3: Effect of Kilovoltage on Film Density

Increased kilovoltage
(Large paper clip)

Decreased kilovoltage
(Small paper clip)

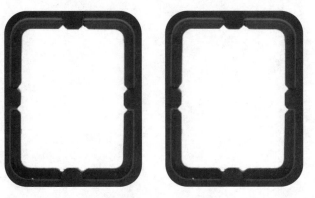

Record the technique settings used for this exercise below.

Increased kilovoltage:
mA _____
kVp_____
impulses _____

Decreased kilovoltage:
mA _____
kVp _____
impulses _____

Part 4: Effect of Kilovoltage on Film Contrast

Increased kilovoltage
(Large paper clip)

Decreased kilovoltage
(Small paper clip)

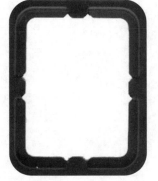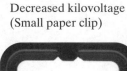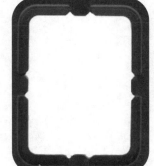

Record the technique settings used for this exercise below.

Increased kilovoltage:
mA _____
kVp_____
impulses _____

Decreased kilovoltage:
mA _____
kVp _____
impulses _____

Part 5: Effect of Film Speed on Film Density

"F" speed film
Increased film speed
(No paper clip)

"D" speed film
Decreased kilovoltage
(Small paper clip)

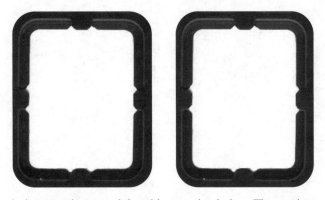

Record the technique settings used for this exercise below. The settings should be the same for both "F" and "D" speed film exposures. The film speed is the variable in this exercise.

Film speeds "F" and "D":
mA _____
kVp _____
impulses _____

Part 6: Effect of PID Length and the Inverse Square Law on Film Density

16″ PID
Standard settings
(No paper clip)

8″ PID
Unchanged settings
(Large paper clip)

8″ PID
Decreased impulse time
(Small paper clip)

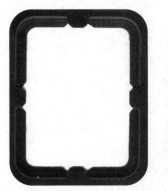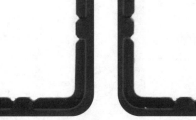

Record the technique settings used for this exercise below. The settings should be the same for both the 16″ PID with standard setting and the 8″ PID with unchanged settings.

16″ and 8″ PID
Standard and Unchanged settings
mA _____
kVp _____
impulses _____

8″ PID
Decreased exposure time
mA _____
kVp _____
impulses _____

Exposure Variables—Factors Affecting the Radiographic Image **231**

Procedure 9.1

Instructions for Assembling a Step Wedge

Varying the thickness or density of an object can vary the amount of radiation reaching the film. A step wedge is constructed of a radiopaque material arranged to vary in thickness from decreased density to increased density. Follow these instructions to assemble a step wedge to use to demonstrate the effect of changing the kVp setting on image contrast. Compare your step wedge with the one pictured in Figure 9.5 ■.

1. Obtain six sheets of lead foil from intraoral film packets.
2. Assemble three piles of two lead foil sheets each.
3. Layer each of the three piles into "steps" of increasing thickness
4. Tape securely together.

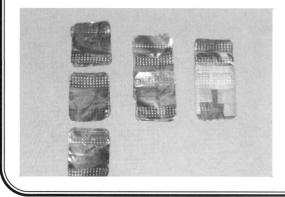

Figure 9.5 *Left:* six sheets of lead foil assembled into three piles of two sheets each; *Middle:* each of the three piles have been layered into "steps" of increasing thickness; *Right:* finished step wedge secured with tape.

I. Visual characteristics of the radiographic image
   A. Density
      1. Overall darkness of the image
      2. Related to the amount of silver within the film emulsion
   B. Contrast (Figure 9.6 ■)
      1. Differences in densities between various regions of the image
      2. High contrast
         a. Very dark areas and very light areas, little shade gradient in between
         b. Also referred to as short scale
      3. Low contrast
         a. Relatively dark and light areas, with many shade gradients in between
         b. Also referred to as long scale
   C. Resolution
      1. Ability of the image to separate close structures or precisely define an edge or outline of a structure
      2. Also referred to as sharpness, clarity, definition, graininess, mottle, noise
   D. Magnification
      1. The degree to which the image represents the actual size of the structure
      2. Creates a fuzzy image edge or penumbra
   E. Distortion
      1. Unequal magnification of the image
      2. Image is not an actual representation of the structure
   F. Radiopaque
      1. Light gray to white or clear areas of the film image
      2. Represents dense objects not easily penetrated by the x-ray beam
   G. Radiolucent
      1. Dark gray to black areas of the film image
      2. Represents less dense objects easily penetrated by the x-ray beam

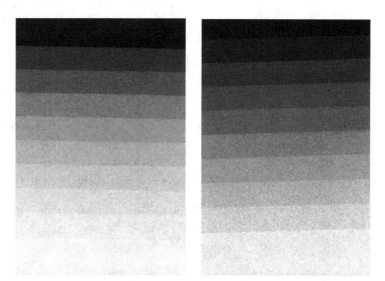

Figure 9.6 *Left:* high contrast (short scale) image produced with 70 kVp; *Right:* low contrast (long scale) image produced with 90 kVp.

Exposure Variables—Factors Affecting the Radiographic Image   **235**

II. X-ray beam factors that affect the radiographic image
- A. Milliamperage (mA)
  1. Controls the amount of radiation reaching the film
  2. Directly proportional to film density
     - a. Increased mA results in increased film density
     - b. Decreased mA results in decreased film density
- B. Kilovoltage (kVp)
  1. Controls the penetrating power of the x-ray beam
  2. Directly proportional to the film density
     - a. Increased penetration of the x-ray beam results in more x-ray photons reaching the film.
     - b. Decreased penetration of the x-ray beam results in less x-ray photons reaching the film.
  3. Inversely proportional to the film contrast
     - a. Increased penetration of the x-ray beam results in lower image contrast.
     - b. Decreased penetration of the x-ray beam results in higher image contrast.
- C. Exposure time (impulses)
  1. Controls the length of time the patient is exposed to the set mA and kVp conditions
  2. Directly proportional to the film density
     - a. Increased exposure time results in more x-ray photons reaching the film.
     - b. Decreased exposure time results in less x-ray photons reaching the film.
- D. Filtration
  1. Controls the amount and penetrating strength of radiation reaching the film
  2. Inversely proportional to the film density
     - a. Increased filtration of the x-ray beam results in lower image density.
     - b. Decreased filtration of the x-ray beam results in higher image density.
- E. Collimation
  1. Controls the amount of radiation reaching the film by restricting the size and shape of the x-ray beam
  2. Inversely proportional to the film density
     - a. Increased collimation of the x-ray beam results in lower image density through reduced film fog.
     - b. Decreased collimation of the x-ray beam results in higher image density through increased film fog.
  3. Inversely proportional to the film contrast
     - a. Increased collimation of the x-ray beam results in higher image contrast through reduced film fog.
     - b. Decreased collimation of the x-ray beam results in lower image contrast through increased film fog.

III. Film factors that affect the radiographic image
- A. Silver halide crystal amount
  1. Controls film speed

2. Directly proportional to the number of crystals present within the emulsion
   a. Increased crystal amount increases film speed.
   b. Decreased crystal amount decreases film speed.
3. Faster speed film requires less radiation to record an image
4. Directly proportional to the film density
   a. Increased film speed results in increased film density.
   b. Decreased film speed results in decreased film density.

B. Silver halide crystal size
1. Controls film speed
2. Directly proportional to the size of the crystals within the emulsion
   a. Increased crystal size increases film speed.
   b. Decreased crystal size decreases film speed.
3. Faster speed film requires less radiation to record an image.
4. Directly proportional to the film density
   a. Increased film speed results in increased film density.
   b. Decreased film speed results in decreased film density.
5. Controls the image resolution
6. Inversely proportional to the size of crystals within the emulsion
   a. Increased crystal size decreases image resolution.
   b. Decreased crystal size increases image resolution.

IV. Subject/object factors that affect the radiographic image
A. Subject thickness
1. Patient size varies
   a. Child
   b. Average adult
   c. Obesity
2. Patient density varies
   a. Edentulous
   b. Less dense bone structure
   c. Dense bone structure
3. Controls the amount of radiation reaching the film by attenuating (stopping) all or a portion of the x-rays
4. Inversely proportional to the film density
   a. Increased patient-subject thickness or density results in lower image density
   b. Decreased patient-subject thickness or density results in higher image density

B. Object density
1. Hard tissue
   a. Enamel
   b. Dentin
   c. Cementum
   d. Bone
2. Soft tissue
   a. Skin (lips, nose, cheek)
   b. Fat
   c. Air
3. Controls the amount of radiation reaching the film by attenuating (stopping) all or a portion of the x-rays

4. Inversely proportional to the film density
   a. Increased object thickness, density, or atomic number results in lower image density
   b. Decreased object thickness, density, or atomic number results in higher image density

V. Geometric factors that affect radiographic image
   A. Controls the image magnification, distortion, and resolution
   B. Shadow cast principles. Geometric distortion is decreased by:
      1. Decreasing the size of the focal spot
      2. Increasing the target-to-film distance
      3. Decreasing the object-to-film distance
      4. Aligning the plane of the film packet parallel to the long axis of the tooth
      5. Directing the central ray of the x-ray beam perpendicular to both the film plane and the long axis of the tooth

VI. Interrelated actions on the factors affecting the radiographic image
   A. Milliamperage
      1. Change the mA (milliamperage) setting when more or less radiation is desired.
         a. More radiation may be desired when a shorter exposure time is necessary.
         b. Example: Patient with slight tremors preventing a still subject.
         c. Lower mA reduces the size of the focal spot by concentrating the electron beam at a smaller point.
      2. A change in mA requires a counter change in the exposure time to obtain an image of similar density.
         a. The sum of the mA plus the exposure time in seconds equals the mAs (milliamperage seconds).
         b. The mAs product must be equal to obtain similar image density.
         c. Example: 10 mA + 0.6 seconds = 6 mAs
                     15 mA + 0.4 seconds = 6 mAs
   B. Kilovoltage
      1. Change the kilovoltage setting when more or less penetration of the x-ray beam is desired.
         a. Increasing the kVp (kilovoltage) may be desired for a decreased image contrast.
         b. Example: Subtle periodontal changes may appear more distinctly when kVp is increased.
         c. Decreasing the kVp (kilovoltage) may be desired for an increased image contrast.
         d. Example: Proximal surface caries detection may be enhanced with a decreased kVp (kilovoltage).
      2. A change in the kVp requires a counter change in the exposure time to obtain an image of similar density.
         a. When increasing the kVp by 15, decrease the exposure time by one-half.
         b. When decreasing the kVp by 15, increase the exposure time by one-half.

C. Exposure time
   1. Change the exposure time when more or less radiation is desired.
      a. Child patient: decrease the exposure time by one-half (for children under age 10) to one-third (children aged 10–15) that recommended for adult patients
      b. Edentulous patients: one-third the exposure time recommended for dentulous patients
      c. Anterior radiographs: one-fifth the exposure time recommended for posterior radiographs
      d. Suspected impacted maxillary third molars: one impulse setting over the recommended setting for the standard maxillary molar periapical
   2. A change in the exposure time is not usually accompanied by a counter change in any other technique variable. Instead, the change in exposure time is considered a counter change in response to the above subject/object variables to obtain an image of similar density.
D. Film speed
   1. Change the film speed when more or less radiation is desired.
      a. Increasing the film speed (from "D" speed to "E" or "F" speed) may be desired for a lower patient radiation dose.
      b. Some clinicians have a preference for viewing the visual image obtained with "D" speed film.
   2. A change in the film speed requires a counter change in the exposure time to obtain an image of similar density.
      a. When increasing the film speed from "D" to "E" speed, decrease the exposure time by one-half.
      b. When decreasing the film speed from "E" to "D" speed, increase the exposure time by one-half.
      c. When increasing the film speed from "E" to "F" speed, decrease the exposure time by 20 percent.
      d. When decreasing the film speed from "F" to "E" speed, increase the exposure time by 20 percent.
E. PID length
   1. Change the PID length when accurate image representation is desired.
      a. Increasing the PID length (from 8″ to 12″ or 16″) may be desired for improved image clarity.
      b. Decreasing the PID length (from 16″ or 12″ to 8″) may be desired for ease of aligning the tube head into position.
      c. Example: The bisecting technique requires increased vertical angulation over the paralleling technique. This increased angulation may be difficult to achieve with the longer PID Small operatories with limited working space may make the 16″ PID cumbersome.
   2. A change in PID length requires a counter change in the exposure time to obtain an image of similar density.
      a. When increasing the PID length (from 8″ to 12″ or 16″), increase the exposure time.

b. When decreasing the PID length (from 16″ or 12″ to 8″), decrease the exposure time.
3. Utilize the inverse square law to calculate the required exposure time when changing the PID length
   a. The intensity of the x-radiation is inversely proportional to the square of the distance from the source of x-radiation to the object.
   b. Formula for calculating the intensity of the x-ray beam when changing PID length:

$$\frac{\text{Original Intensity}}{\text{New Intensity}} = \frac{\text{New Distance}^2}{\text{Original Distance}^2}$$

   c. The exposure time is directly proportional to the square of the distance from the source of x-radiation to the object
   d. Formula for calculating the exposure time adjustment when changing the PID length:

$$\frac{\text{Original Exposure Time}}{\text{New Exposure Time}} = \frac{\text{Original Distance}^2}{\text{New Distance}^2}$$

   e. General rule of thumb: when increasing the distance by 2, increase the exposure time by 4. When reducing the distance by 2, decrease the exposure time by 4.

BIBLIOGRAPHY

ADA Council on Scientific Affairs. An update on radiographic practices:information and recommendations. *Journal of the American Dental Association.* 2001;132:234–238.

Frommer, HH, Stabulas-Savage, JJ. *Radiology for the Dental Professional.* 8th ed. St. Louis, MO: Elsevier Mosby; 2005:41–56.

Haring, JI, Howerton, LJ. *Dental Radiography. Principles and Techniques,* 3rd ed. St. Louis, MO: Elsevier; 2006:28–35, 89–97.

Johnson, ON, Thomson, EM. *Essentials of Dental Radiography for Dental Assistants and Hygienists,* 8th ed. Upper Saddle River, NJ: Prentice Hall; 2007:35–48.

Olson, SS. *Dental Radiography Laboratory Manual.* Philadelphia, PA: WB Saunders Co.; 1995:32–47.

Thomson, EM, Tolle L. A practical guide for using radiographs in the assessment of periodontal disease. Part I: technique. *Practical Hygiene,* 1994;3(1):11–16.

White, SC, Pharoah, MJ. *Oral Radiology. Principles and Interpretation,* 5th ed. St. Louis, MO: Elsevier, 2004:13–16.

Refer to the experiments in parts 1 through 6 of this exercise to answer the following questions.

1. With all other exposure settings remaining constant, an INCREASE IN EXPOSURE TIME will result in:
   - A. Increased film density
   - B. Decreased film density

2. With all other exposure settings remaining constant, a DECREASE IN EXPOSURE TIME will result in:
   - A. Increased film density
   - B. Decreased film density

3. With all other exposure settings remaining constant, a DECREASE IN MILLIAMPERAGE will result in:
   - A. Increased film density
   - B. Decreased film density

4. With all other exposure settings remaining constant, a DECREASE IN KILOVOLTAGE will result in:
   - A. Increased film density
   - B. Decreased film density

5. With all other exposure settings remaining constant, a DECREASE IN KILOVOLTAGE will result in:
   - A. Increased film contrast
   - B. Decreased film contrast

6. With all other exposure settings remaining constant, a DECREASE IN FILM SPEED will result in:
   - A. Increased film density
   - B. Decreased film density

7. With all other exposure settings remaining constant, a DECREASE IN PID LENGTH will result in:
   - A. Increased film density
   - B. Decreased film density

8. With a 16″ PID, an exposure intensity is 100 mSv. With all other exposure settings remaining constant, what would the intensity be if an 8″ PID is used?
   - A. 400 mSv
   - B. 200 mSv
   - C. 50 mSv
   - D. 25 mSv

9. You work in a dental practice that uses an 8″ PID with an exposure time of 12 impulses. The dentist retires, and the new dentist who buys his practice asks you to stay on and work with her. One of the things she changes is the PID length to 16″. What will you do to the impulse timer setting to compensate for this change?
   - A. Reduce the exposure time to 3 impulses.
   - B. Reduce the exposure time to 6 impulses.
   - C. Increase the exposure time to 24 impulses.
   - D. Increase the exposure time to 48 impulses.

10. Indicate how you determined the answers to questions 8 and 9 by utilizing the Inverse Square Law.

Demonstrate how you arrived at the answer to question 8 by working the following formula:

The intensity of the x-radiation is inversely proportional to the square of the distance from the source of x-radiation to the object.

$$\frac{\text{Original Intensity}}{\text{New Intensity}} = \frac{\text{New Distance}^2}{\text{Original Distance}^2}$$

Demonstrate how you arrived at the answer to question 9 by working the following formula:

The exposure time is directly proportional to the square of the distance from the source of x-radiation to the object.

$$\frac{\text{Original Exposure Time}}{\text{New Exposure Time}} = \frac{\text{Original Distance}^2}{\text{New Distance}^2}$$

_____

_____

_____

_____

_____

_____

_____

_____

_____

_____

Identifying and Correcting Radiographic Errors

INTRODUCTION

Dental radiographs play a valuable role in the assessment and diagnosis of oral conditions. However, regardless of value, it is important to understand that radiation exposure carries a risk of biological harm. Exposure to dental radiation should therefore be kept to a minimum. The greatest contributor to excess patient radiation exposure is retake radiographs. Retake radiographs are needed when errors are made that compromise radiographic quality. Retake radiographs double patient exposure; increase the radiation dose to the same tissue area; increase the dose rate, since most retakes are taken without a recovery period between exposures; require additional patient consent; reduce patient confidence in the oral health care professional's ability to provide care; and decrease productivity. Additionally, errors that do not result in retakes still diminish the usefulness of the radiograph. Images that lack proper density, contrast, and clarity reduce the value of the radiograph and jeopardize diagnosis. Reduced quality radiographs are also a practice management risk should they be required as evidence in legal matters.

Radiographic errors can be organized into three categories: technique errors, processing errors, and film handling errors. Errors may be made singly or as a result of a combination of errors. Often a technique error may mimic a processing error and vice versa. Awareness of the more common errors can help the radiographer take steps to prevent the errors from occurring in the first place. Recognition of radiographic pitfalls will also help the radiographer to evaluate radiographic images for quality. And, most important, knowledge of the cause of the error and its corrective action will aid the radiographer in taking the appropriate steps to prevent additional retake radiographs.

The purpose of this exercise is to allow the student to create radiographic errors. By creating the error, the student is given the opportunity to study the error's cause and corrective action. Additionally, students will be given the opportunity to identify radiographic pitfalls and to develop the problem-solving skills necessary to recommend the appropriate corrective action.

OBJECTIVES

Following completion of this lab activity, you will be able to:

1. Identify characteristics of a quality radiographic image.

2. Recognize common radiographic technique, processing, and film handling errors.

3. Recommend appropriate corrective action when confronted with a poor quality radiograph.

MATERIALS

Teaching manikin or skull

Lead (or lead equivalent) apron and thyroid collar

Size #1 and size #2 radiographic films

Periapical and bitewing film holders

Cotton-tipped applicators

Viewbox

PREPARATION

1. Study the chapter outline to prepare for this laboratory exercise. An understanding of the material presented in the outline is required to complete this activity.

2. Prepare radiology operatory. Set up teaching manikin or skull. Ensure that correct "patient" positioning is achieved, that is, occlusal plane parallel to the floor, midsagittal plane perpendicular to the floor.

3. Place lead apron (or lead-equivalent barrier) and thyroid collar over the "patient."

4. Instructor demonstration may enhance knowledge of the laboratory exercise.

LABORATORY EXERCISE ACTIVITIES

Part 1: Technique Error—Comparing Accidental White Light Exposure and No Exposure Errors

The most basic skill of radiographic error identification is being able to determine if a radiographic film has been overexposed, as is the case when a film is accidentally exposed to white light or not exposed at all. The ability to distinguish between which error causes the radiographic image to be too dark, or black, and which error causes the radiographic image to be too light, or clear, provides the basis for determining more complex errors. The purpose of this activity is to allow the radiographer to purposely produce these two errors and then to present the challenge to determine which is which.

1. Obtain two size #2 films.

2. **DO NOT EXPOSE THESE FILMS TO RADIATION.**

3. Go to the darkroom, secure the door, turn off the overhead white light, and turn on the safelight.

4. Open and process one of the films in the usual manner.

5. Next, turn on the overhead white light and open and process the other film under *unsafe* white light conditions.

Part 2: Technique Error—Demonstration of Reversed Film Error

There are several errors that can cause a radiographic image to appear too light or underexposed. Prior to taking corrective action, the cause of the light image should be determined. Without determining the cause of the error, inappropriate corrective action may result in a repeat error. Therefore, the first step in determining the cause of a light image is to view the film carefully for the image of the pattern embossed into the lead foil of the film packet. The purpose of this activity is to demonstrate how this pattern gets imaged onto the radiograph when the film packet is positioned into the oral cavity backward.

1. Obtain one each of a size #2 and a size #1 radiographic film packet.

2. Prepare to expose the maxillary central incisors periapical radiograph. Place the size #2 film packet in the film-holding device *backward*. Place the film packet so that the printed, colored side is facing the x-ray beam. This is *backward* or *reversed* placement of the film packet.

3. Check posted exposure settings and place and expose the maxillary central incisor periapical radiograph using the paralleling technique.

4. Repeat steps 2 and 3 with the size #1 film packet.

5. Process the two films.

Part 3: Technique Error—Double Exposure Error

One of the most difficult errors for the beginning student to recognize is the double exposure error. This is especially true when the two images are very similar to each other, as is the case when a bitewing radiograph is double exposed with another bitewing radiograph of a different region. The purpose of this activity is to provide the radiographer with the opportunity to view the unique image that results from a double exposure error.

1. Obtain one size #2 radiographic film packet.

2. Prepare to expose the right premolar and the right molar bitewing radiographs. Place the film packet in the film-holding device for exposure of the right premolar bitewing radiograph first.

3. Check posted exposure settings and place and expose the right premolar bitewing radiograph.

Identifying and Correcting Radiographic Errors   **245**

4. Next, *using the same film you just exposed,* place the film and film-holding device to expose the right molar bitewing radiograph.

5. Check posted exposure settings and expose the right molar bitewing radiograph.

6. Process the film.

Part 4: Processing Error—Comparison of the Effect of Developer Contamination and Fixer Contamination on Films Prior to Processing

In addition to technique errors, mistakes made in the darkroom can also render a radiograph undiagnostic. Processing errors also result in retake radiographs. The radiographer should possess a working knowledge of the effects processing chemicals have on the radiographic image to be prepared to solve darkroom problems. The purpose of this activity is to simulate the errors that result when attention to darkroom cleanliness is lacking.

1. Obtain two size #2 radiographic film packets.

2. Prepare to expose the maxillary central incisors periapical radiograph. Place the film packets in the film-holding device.

3. Check posted exposure settings, and place and expose the maxillary central incisors periapical radiograph using the paralleling technique, using the first film.

4. Repeat step 3 using the second film.

5. In the darkroom, under safelight conditions, open both film packets, and place the films on a paper towel on the counter.

6. Using a cotton-tipped applicator, place a small drop of developer on one of the films.

7. Obtain a clean cotton-tipped applicator, and place a small drop of fixer on the other film (Figure 10.1 ■).

8. Wait approximately 1 minute and then process the films as usual.

Part 5: Processing Error—Inadequate Fixation

The radiographer should possess the ability to identify when the processing chemicals are not functioning at peak potential. To develop this skill, a working knowledge of the function of each chemical is needed. The purpose

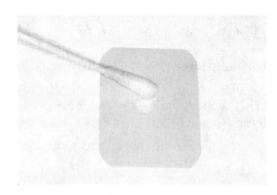

Figure 10.1 Using a cotton-tipped applicator to apply a small drop of fixer to the film prior to processing.

of this activity is to demonstrate the effect of inadequate fixation time on the resultant radiographic image.

1. Obtain one size #2 radiographic film packet.
2. Prepare to expose the maxillary central incisor periapical radiograph. Place the film packet in the film-holding device.
3. Check posted exposure settings and place and expose the maxillary central incisor periapical radiograph using the paralleling technique.
4. Process the film. *However, reduce the fixer time to only one-fourth of the standard time.*

Part 6: Processing Error—Fixer First Error

Whether processing manually or utilizing an automatic film processor, the steps for film processing must be performed in order. The developer and the fixer play a specific role in the processing procedure. Reversing the procedure order can create disastrous effects. The purpose of this activity is to demonstrate the effect of placing the exposed radiographic film into the fixer first during manual processing and/or incorrectly filling the first compartment of an automatic processor with fixer instead of developer.

1. Obtain one size #2 radiographic film packet.
2. Prepare to expose the maxillary central incisor periapical radiograph. Place the film packet in the film-holding device.
3. Check posted exposure settings, and place and expose the maxillary central incisor periapical radiograph using the paralleling technique.
4. Process the film by placing it *into the fixer first.*

Part 7: Film Handling Error—Bending the Film Packet Prior to Exposure

Careful film handling is needed to avoid bending or creasing the film packet when loading it into a film holder prior to exposure. The purpose of this activity is to demonstrate what effect bending the film will have on the resultant image. Awareness of this result may also help the radiographer understand why film bending to fit the oral cavity is contraindicated.

1. Obtain one size #2 radiographic film packet.
2. Prepare to expose the maxillary central incisor periapical radiograph. *Prior to placing the film packet in the film-holding device, crease one corner of the film packet.*
3. Check posted exposure settings and place and expose the maxillary central incisor periapical radiograph using the paralleling technique.
4. Process the film.

Part 8: A Problem-Solving Activity

For the past several weeks you have been practicing intraoral radiographic techniques for the first time. As a beginning radiographer, you have probably created some errors along the way. This is your chance to use these "mistakes" as a valuable teaching tool. Choose one of your radiographic errors and mount this film on p. 253. Submit this error film page to your instructor who will number and post one error page from everyone in the class. The challenge to you will be to view each of the posted errors and (1) identify the cause and (2) suggest a corrective action. If you do not have an error to submit for this activity, purposely create one now. Use the outline that follows to select an error to create.

COMPETENCY AND EVALUATION

1. Mount the processed films on the simulated film mount pages that follow. Secure with a piece of tape placed along the top edge of the film only, so that the films may be raised slightly, to allow light underneath for ease of viewing. The use of removable transparent tape will allow the film mount page to be used more than once.

   NOTE: Use the labial mounting method. (See Laboratory Exercise 8, Film Mounting and Radiographic Landmarks, for details.) The raised portion of the embossed dot is toward you (convex) when placing the film onto the page.

2. Examine the resultant radiographic images in each of the first seven parts of this exercise. Based on your results, summarize the following in your own words:

   a. How would you explain the effect of accidental white light exposure compared with no exposure of the film? Why is one dark and the other clear?

   b. How can you tell when the film packet has been placed in the patient's mouth backward?

   c. Describe the unique appearance of accidentally exposing the same film twice.

   d. Describe the effects of developer and fixer contamination prior to developing exposed films. Why does one cause dark radiolucent artifacts while the other causes clear, white, or radiopaque artifacts?

   e. Describe the effect of inadequate fixation.

   f. Describe the effect of placing the film into the fixer solution first.

   g. What effect will bending the film have on the resultant image?

3. When your instructor has posted the errors collected from your class, view each of the samples and write out your answer to the these questions:

   a. What is the error created here?

   b. What is the corrective action?

   NOTE: Your answers should be technical and not obvious. For example, do not answer "blank film" for a radiograph that is clear. "No exposure" or "unexposed" would be a more appropriate answer. Likewise, do not answer "expose the film" as the obvious corrective action. Think about how the film could have resulted in no exposure. It is possible that the film did not get exposed because the radiographer mixed up the exposed film packets with the unexposed film packets while taking a full mouth series. Hence, a more appropriate answer for the corrective action would be "follow an organized and systematic method of exposing film packets during the radiographic procedure."

There may be more than one correct answer for each error. In our example above, we suggested a technique error for the clear or blank film. A clear film could also result from the processing error of placing the film in the fixer first. Again, your corrective action should not state the obvious, "place the film in the developer first." Instead, think about how this error could have resulted. A more appropriate response would be "label the processing chemical tanks," to prevent placing the film into the fixer first.

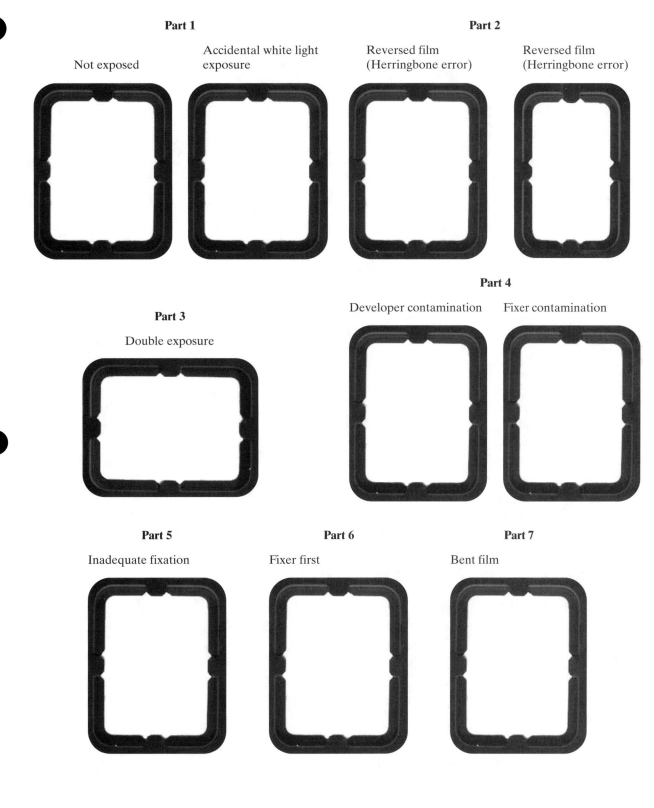

Part 1

Not exposed

Accidental white light exposure

Part 2

Reversed film (Herringbone error)

Reversed film (Herringbone error)

Part 3

Double exposure

Part 4

Developer contamination

Fixer contamination

Part 5

Inadequate fixation

Part 6

Fixer first

Part 7

Bent film

Part 8

Error Identification

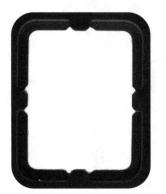

Submit this error page to your instructor to number and post for part 8 of this exercise.

I. Characteristics of diagnostic quality dental radiographs
  A. General characteristics
    1. Image is an accurate representation of the area being radio-graphed.
    2. Exhibits correct density (not too light/too dark).
    3. Free of image distortion (magnification/elongation/foreshort-ening).
    4. No overlapping of the interproximal areas.
    5. No cone-cut error.
    6. Free of technical, processing, and film handling errors.
  B. Bitewing radiographs
    1. Correct teeth are imaged.
      a. Anterior bitewing film packet placement
        1) Central incisors bitewing radiograph should image the maxillary and mandibular central and lateral incisors, centered in the middle of the film; if using a size #2 film, the mesial edges of the right and left canines should be imaged.
        2) Canine bitewing radiograph should image the maxillary and mandibular canines, centered in the middle of the image, and as much of the first premolar and the lateral incisor as possible.
        3) Premolar bitewing radiograph should image the distal portion of the maxillary and mandibular canines, entire maxillary and mandibular first and second premolars, entire maxillary and mandibular first molars, and the mesial portion of the maxillary and mandibular second molars.
        4) Molar bitewing radiograph should image the distal portion of the maxillary and mandibular second premolars and the entire maxillary and mandibular first, second, and third (if present) molars.
    2. Equal representation of the maxillary and mandibular arches is imaged.
    3. The occlusal plane is straight or slightly curved upward.
    4. The most distal contact is imaged (third molars if erupted).
  C. Periapical radiographs
    1. Correct teeth are imaged.
      a. Anterior periapical film packet placement may vary among practices. The following is one example of accurate film packet placement for imaging the anterior teeth (See Exercise 3, Periapical Radiographs—Paralleling Techniques, for additional acceptable film packet placements):
        1) Central incisors periapical radiograph should image the entire central and lateral incisors, centered in the middle of the film; if using a size #2 film, the mesial edges of the right and left canines should be imaged.
        2) Canine periapical radiograph should image the entire canine, centered in the middle of the image, and as much of the first premolar and the lateral incisor as possible.

b. Posterior periapical film packet placement is the same for most practices.
   1) Premolar periapical radiograph should image the distal portion of the canine, entire first and second premolars, first molar, and a mesial portion of the second molar.
   2) Molar periapical radiograph should image the distal portion of the second premolar, entire first, second, and third (if present) molars.
2. Image at least 2 mm of alveolar bone beyond the apices of the teeth being imaged.
3. One-eighth to one-fourth inch margin present between the edge of the film and the crowns of the teeth being imaged.
4. Each tooth is imaged at least once, preferably twice in a full mouth series of periapical radiographs.
5. The embossed dot should be positioned at the incisal/occlusal edge of the film.

II. Radiographic errors
   A. Dark film
      1. Results from overexposure
         a. Error
            1) Increased exposure time impulse setting
            2) Increased milliamperage setting
            3) Increased kilovoltage setting
            4) Accidental white light exposure
         b. Corrective action
            1) Post exposure setting chart for reference.
            2) Consult the exposure setting chart prior to each exposure.
            3) Adjust the exposure settings based on the thickness/density of the subject/object being imaged.
            4) Locate the overhead white light switch away from the working area to prevent accidentally turning on the white light.
      2. Results from overdeveloping
         a. Error
            1) Increased time in the developing solution
            2) Increased developer temperature
            3) Overconcentrated chemical mix
            4) Contaminating the developer solution with fixer chemistry
         b. Corrective action
            1) Consult the time/temperature chart prior to manually processing films.
            2) Adjust the time/temperature prior to automatically processing films.
            3) Take the temperature of the developer prior to manually processing films.
            4) Secure the developer thermostat in the automatic processing unit.
            5) Carefully mix concentrated chemicals with the appropriate ratio of water prior to use.

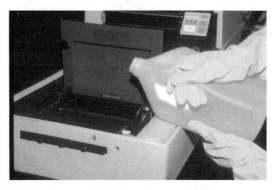

Figure 10.2 Separating the developer and fixer chemicals during replenishing helps to avoid chemical contamination that can result in poor quality radiographs.

      6) Handle replenishing chemicals carefully to avoid contamination. (See Figure 1.2 and Figure 10.2 ■.)

B. Partially dark films/black artifacts

  1. Results from overexposure

    a. Error

      1) Accidental light leak

      2) Static electricity exposure

    b. Corrective action

      1) Carefully remove film packet from the film-holding device so as not to tear the outer protective wrap, allowing white light to enter the film packet and expose the film.

      2) Allow the film to completely enter the automatic processor prior to turning on the white light.

      3) Secure the light-tight cover of the manual processing tanks prior to turning on the white light.

      4) Slowly unwrap film packets to avoid creating a static discharge of white light.

      5) Utilize a humidifier to reduce dry conditions conducive to static electricity.

      6) Place an antistatic treated grounding device in the darkroom such as commercially available antistatic sprays or clothes dryer fabric sheets to discharge static prior to film handling.

  2. Results from overdeveloping

    a. Error

      1) Developer contamination

      2) Overlapped films during processing (fixer not in contact with film emulsion)

      3) Roller marks

    b. Corrective action

      1) Maintain cleanliness in the darkroom to avoid chemical contamination of films prior to processing.

      2) When loading films into the automatic processor, use alternating feeder slots or wait approximately 5–10 seconds between each film to avoid overlapping films; if fixer does not contact the emulsion, that portion of the film will fade to black when removed from the processor and exposed to white light.

3) Do not overload manual processing tanks with several film processing racks to avoid film contact.

4) Properly maintain processor, replenishing and replacing chemistry according to manufacturer's recommendations.

a) As exhausted chemistry breaks down, the solutions become "slick," causing films to become "stuck" on the automatic processing rollers.

b) As the rollers turn, the films do not advance, but "slide" on the turning rollers, which create black horizontal bands of "overdeveloped" areas on the films.

3. Results from film handling

a. Error

1) Film bending/creasing

2) Embossed dot wrongly positioned during packet placement in the oral cavity (Figure 10.3 ■)

3) Black paper stuck to the film emulsion

4) Glove powder contamination

b. Corrective action

1) Carefully handle films, especially when placing film into film holders, to avoid bending or cracking the film emulsion.

2) Use an edge cushion or smaller sized film to ease placement intraorally, rather than bend or crease a large film to fit the oral cavity.

3) Place the embossed dot away from the area of interest, i.e., place at the occlusal/incisal when placing the film for periapical radiographs.

4) Immediately upon removal from the oral cavity, wipe excess saliva from the film packet (especially paper wrapped packets) to prevent saliva from seeping into the packet causing the black paper to adhere to the film. (See Figure 6.2.)

5) Carefully unwrap film packets, to completely separate the film from the outer plastic/paper wrap, the black paper insert, and the lead foil sheet.

6) Follow infection control protocol to avoid touching the unprocessed films with gloves or hands contaminated with glove powder residue. (See Laboratory Exercise 6, Infection Control and Student Partner Practice.)

C. Light film

1. Results from underexposure

a. Error

1) Decreased exposure time impulse setting.

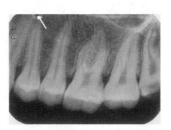

Figure 10.3 When placed near the area of interest such as the apex of the tooth, the embossed dot may obscure pertinent diagnostic information.

2) Decreased milliamperage setting.

3) Decreased kilovoltage setting.

4) Distance between the open end of the PID and the patient's skin was increased (Figure 10.4 ■).

5) Backward placement of the film packet intraorally so that the x-ray beam must penetrate the lead foil prior to reaching the film.

    a) Placing the film packet so that the colored side with the printed information is facing the x-ray beam (Figure 10.5 ■)

    b) Lack of knowledge about which is the front side of the film packet

    c) Hurried, unorganized film packet placement

    d) Utilizing an unfamiliar film-holding device

b. Corrective action

1) Check for a reversed film packet placement as evidenced by the presence of a tire-track or block pattern imaged on to the film (Figure 10.6 ■). Sometimes referred to as herringbone error after the herringbone pattern produced by early commercial film products.

    a) When in doubt about the correct side of the film packet, read the information written on the colored

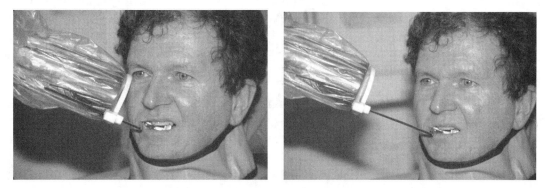

Figure 10.4 The photo on the left demonstrates the correct position of the PID and the external aiming device of the film holder. The position of the PID and external aiming device of the film holder in the photo on the right would result in an underexposed radiographic image.

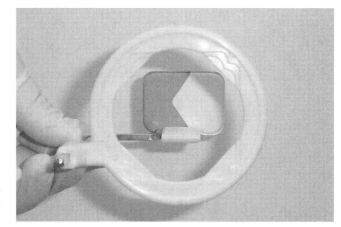

Figure 10.5 Backward film packet placement. Note that the back of the film packet will be incorrectly exposed first, resulting in a light image.

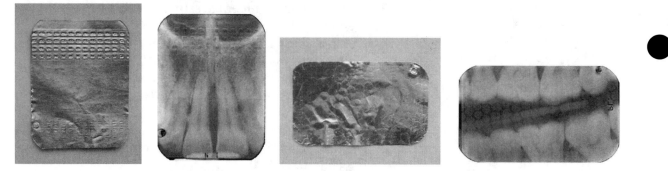

Figure 10.6 These embossed patterns will be imaged when the lead foil faces the x-ray beam, resulting in "herringbone" error. Note the different patterns, depending on the film size and manufacturer.

side. The statement "opposite side toward tube" or similar wording will guide you.
   b) Be systematic and organized when placing and exposing radiographs.
   c) Become familiar with the film-holding device before using it to avoid placing the film incorrectly.
2) Post exposure setting chart near the x-ray unit control panel for reference.
3) Consult the exposure setting chart prior to each exposure.
4) Adjust the exposure settings based on the thickness/density of the subject/object being imaged.
5) Keep the exposure button depressed throughout the duration of the exposure.
6) Place the open end of the PID as close to the patient's skin as possible without touching; if using a film holder with an external aiming device, slide the aiming device in toward the patient, until it almost contacts the skin (Figure 10.4).

2. Results from underdeveloping
   a. Error
      1) Decreased time in the developing solution
      2) Decreased developer temperature
      3) Underconcentrated chemical mix
      4) Exhausted chemicals
   b. Corrective action
      1) Consult the time/temperature chart prior to manually processing films.
      2) Adjust the time/temperature prior to automatically processing films.
      3) Check the temperature of the developer prior to manually processing films.
      4) Check fluid level of the developer in the automatic processor to ensure that the films will be submerged throughout the processing procedure.
      5) Carefully mix concentrated chemicals with the appropriate ratio of water prior to use.

6) Replenish and change chemistry according to manufacturer's recommendations.
D. Clear/blank film
   1. Results from no exposure (unexposed film)
      a. Error
         1) Confusing the film with one that had been exposed
         2) Not turning on the power to the x-ray unit
         3) Placing the film packet, but neglecting to align the PID toward the film
      b. Corrective action
         1) Develop a systematic routine for exposing radiographs.
         2) Label exposed films and keep separated from unexposed films during the procedure.
         3) Follow an organized and systematic routine; perform pre-alignment of the PID prior to placing the film packet intraorally.
   2. Results from incorrect processing
      a. Error
         1) Placing the film into the fixer solution first, allowing the fixer to remove the undeveloped silver halide crystals from the emulsion
         2) Automatically processing the film with no developer solution in the tank
         3) Extended time in the fixer or water during processing, causing the emulsion to separate from the film base
      b. Corrective action
         1) Label the processing tanks to prevent confusing the developer and fixer tanks.
         2) Read developer and fixer container labels to prevent pouring developer into the fixer tank and fixer into the developing tank during replenishing.
         3) Ensure that the automatic processor is adequately filled with developer solution.
         4) Ensure that the developer tank drain plug is secure to prevent solution from draining out.
         5) Do not leave films overnight in the fixer solution or wash water.
E. Partially clear/blank film/white artifacts
   1. Results from no/underexposure
      a. Error
         1) Cone-cut error
            a) Not centering the film packet in the path of the x-ray beam
            b) Incorrect assembly of the film-holding device, causing the radiographer to center the x-ray beam incorrectly
      b. Corrective action
         1) Use a film-holding device that aids in centering the film in the path of the x-ray beam.
         2) Learn the appropriate assembly of the film-holding device prior to using it.

2. Results from incorrect processing
    a. Error
        1) Fixer contamination of the film prior to processing.
        2) Air bubbles adhering to the film surface during processing.
        3) Overlapped films during processing (developer not in contact with film emulsion).
        4) Attaching a film to the top clip on the manual processing film rack in combination with a reduced developer solution level in the tank (caused by evaporation or extended use) may prevent developer from reaching the top portion of the film; when this film is submerged into the fixer solution, the fixer functions to remove the undeveloped silver halide crystals from the emulsion in this area (Figure 10.7 ■).
    b. Corrective action
        1) Maintain cleanliness in the darkroom to avoid chemical contamination of films prior to processing.
        2) When manually processing, agitate film racks for 5 seconds to remove trapped air bubbles which prevent chemistry from reaching the emulsion.
        3) Do not allow films to contact each other or the sides of the manual processing tanks during processing; if developer does not contact the emulsion, that portion of the film will turn clear/blank when placed into the fixer solution.
        4) Monitor the solution levels.
        5) Replenish solutions regularly.
        6) Do not attach films to the top manual processing film rack.
3. Results from improper film handling and patient management
    a. Error
        1) Foreign object recorded on the film
        2) Scratched emulsion

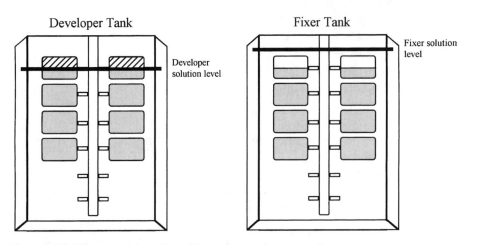

Figure 10.7 When a portion of the film is not developed, the fixer solution functions to remove the undeveloped silver halide crystals from the emulsion, resulting in a clear/bank portion of the radiograph.

3) Crimp mark from film bending prior to exposure
  b. Corrective action
    1) Ask patient to remove metal objects in or near the oral cavity.
      a) Glasses
      b) Partial/full denture
      c) Orthodontic retainer
      d) Facial jewelry (tongue, lip, nose piercing adornments)
    2) Assess the use of the lead thyroid collar for some patients. When used on children or adults with a short neck-to-shoulder relationship, the lead thyroid collar may be in the path of the primary beam.
    3) Carefully handle films, especially when clipping to manual film processing racks, to avoid scratched emulsion.
    4) Avoid overlapping or allowing films to contact each other or the sides of the manual processing tanks to avoid torn emulsion.
    5) Avoid bending the film packet. To increase patient comfort during film packet placement, utilize an edge cushioning product or a smaller size film. (See Laboratory Exercise 7, Patient Management and Student Partner Practice, Figure 7.2.)
F. Green artifacts
  1. Result from incorrect or inadequate film processing
    a. Error
      1) Films become overlapped or stuck together in the automatic processor, preventing chemicals from reaching the emulsion.
      2) Double film packets that are not separated prior to processing prevent chemicals from reaching the emulsion.
      3) Attaching a film to the top clip on the manual processing film rack in combination with a reduced developer and a reduced fixer solution level in both manual processing tanks (caused by evaporation or extended use) may prevent chemicals from reaching a portion of the film. (Figure 10.8 ■)
      4) Weak or exhausted fixer that cannot adequately clear the film.
    b. Corrective action
      1) When loading films into the automatic processor, use alternating feeder slots or wait approximately 5–10 seconds between each film to avoid overlapping, preventing processing chemicals from reaching the film emulsion.
      2) Carefully separate double film packets prior to loading onto manual film processing racks or into the automatic processor.
      3) Monitor the solution levels.
      4) Replenish solutions regularly.
      5) Do not attach films to the top manual processing film rack.

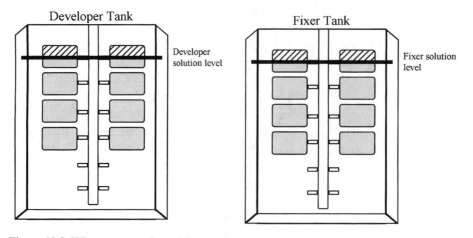

Developer Tank

Developer solution level

Fixer Tank

Fixer solution level

Figure 10.8 When evaporation of chemistry from manual processing tanks prevents both developer and fixer from reaching the film emulsion, the resulting error is a green, unprocessed portion of the film.

G. Brown artifacts
  1. Result from incorrect film processing
    a. Error
      1) Inadequate film rinsing and washing
    b. Corrective action
      1) Allow the films to wash for the full recommended time.
      2) Ensure that the water to the running water bath (for manual processing and the water supply to the automatic processing unit) is turned on.
H. Fogged image
  1. Resulting from overexposure
    a. Error
      1) Inadequate safelighting
      2) Unprotected film use in the operatory
    b. Corrective action
      1) Perform quality assurance tests to determine adequacy of safelighting in the darkroom.
      2) Provide a safe place for films, especially those that were just exposed, away from stray radiation during the radiographic procedure.
  2. Resulting from film handling
    a. Error
      1) Old, expired film
      2) Unprotected film storage
    b. Corrective action
      1) Maintain film inventory that uses the oldest film first.
      2) Provide a safe place for film storage free from heat, humidity, and chemical fumes.
      3) Do not store film in the darkroom.
  3. Results from contaminated solutions
    a. Error
      1) Using the same paddles to stir solutions

2) Not cleaning and drying the manual processing film racks before using again.
3) Careless handling of processing chemistry during replenishment.
4) Switching automatic processor rollers between developer and fixer.
5) Using the same brush or sponge to clean developer and fixer automatic processor rollers or manual processing tanks.

  b. Corrective action
1) Use and maintain separate equipment for developer and fixer.
2) Use care when handling processing chemistry. Cover tanks when not in use.
3) Follow protocol for cleaning and maintaining manual processing film racks and other equipment.
4) Label processing tanks and rollers to maintain separate developer and fixer contact.
5) Label cleaning supplies for use with only the developer or with only the fixer.

I. Damaged film emulsion
  1. Results from reticulation
    a. Error
1) Developing films in extremely hot developer solution and then placing films into extremely cold rinse water causing the emulsion to crack.
2) Improved film and modern processing chemicals lessen the likelihood of producing this error. However, widely varying temperatures of processing solutions may affect the diagnostic quality of the image.

    b. Corrective action
1) Monitor processing solution temperatures.
2) Periodically check the automatic processing solution temperatures manually to confirm settings recommended by manufacturer.
3) Ensure that the automatic processor thermostat is in place at each replenishment/setup.

  2. Results from careless processing
    a. Error
1) Extremely hot processing chemistry may melt or cause a portion or all of the film emulsion to separate from the base.
2) Extended time in the fixer or water during processing, causing the emulsion to separate from the film base.
3) Allowing films to contact each other or the sides of the processing tanks during processing.

    b. Corrective action
1) Monitor processing solution temperatures.
2) Periodically check the automatic processing solution temperatures manually to confirm settings recommended by manufacturer.

3) Ensure that the automatic processor thermostat is in place at each replenishment/setup.
4) Do not leave films overnight in the fixer solution or wash water.
5) Do not overload the manual film-processing tank with several film racks at a time.

J. Technique errors

1. Result from incorrect film packet placement (See Figures 3.14 and 3.15.)
   a. Error
      1) Film packet placement too far anteriorly
      2) Film packet placement too far posteriorly
      3) Film packet placement too far superiorly
      4) Film packet placement too far inferiorly
   b. Corrective action
      1) Examine the patient's oral cavity for mal-aligned, missing, or supernumerary teeth, and adjust film packet placement accordingly.
      2) Possess a working knowledge of which teeth must be imaged on each of the standard periapical and bitewing radiographs included in a full mouth survey.

2. Results in horizontal overlap of the proximal surfaces of the teeth (See Figures 3.18 and 3.19.)
   a. Error
      1) Incorrect horizontal angulation of the x-ray beam
      2) Incorrect film placement in the oral cavity
   b. Corrective action
      1) Align the x-ray beam to intersect the film plane perpendicularly in the horizontal direction. (See Figure 3.10.)
      2) Align the film packet parallel to the teeth being imaged. (See Figure 2.10.)

3. Results in incisal/occlusal edge or apices cut off the image (paralleling technique error)
   a. Error
      1) Incorrect vertical angulation of the x-ray beam
      2) Incorrect film packet placement
   b. Corrective action
      1) The x-ray beam must intersect the film plane perpendicularly in the vertical dimension.
         a) Excessive vertical angulation results in loss of the incisal/occlusal edge imaged. (See Figure 3.16.)
         b) Inadequate vertical angulation results in loss of the apices imaged. (See Figure 3.17.)
      2) Place the film packet parallel to the teeth being imaged.
      3) Direct the patient to close down completely on the bite block of the film holder to ensure recording of the apices of the teeth of interest.
      4) Match the film-holding device with the technique used (paralleling device with the paralleling technique and bisecting device with the bisecting technique).

4. Results in elongation/foreshortening of the image (bisecting technique error)
  a. Error
    1) Incorrect vertical angulation of the x-ray beam
    2) Incorrect film packet placement
    3) Film packet bending
      a) Patient applies too much pressure to film packet while holding in place.
      b) Anatomical structures, such as tori, shallow palatal vault prevent correct film packet placement.
  b. Corrective action
    1) The x-ray beam must intersect the imaginary bisector between the film plane and the long axis of the tooth perpendicularly in the vertical dimension.
      a) Excessive vertical angulation results in foreshortening of the image. (See Figure 4.17)
      b) Inadequate vertical angulation results in elongation of the image. (See Figure 4.18)
    2) Place the film packet as close to the teeth being imaged as possible without bending.
    3) Inspect the patient's oral cavity for possible obstructions in film packet placement and make adjustments as needed. (See Laboratory Exercise 7, Patient Management and Student Partner Practice.)
    4) Direct the patient to close down completely on the bite block of the film holder to ensure recording of the apices of the teeth of interest.
    5) Match the film-holding device with the technique used (paralleling device with the paralleling technique and bisecting device with the bisecting technique).
    6) Do not utilize the patient's finger as a film-holding device.
5. Results in blurred image
  a. Error
    1) Patient movement
    2) Film packet movement
    3) PID/tube head movement
  b. Corrective action
    1) Establish good patient rapport to obtain maximum cooperation during the radiographic procedure
    2) Educate the patient to the role they play in obtaining quality radiographs
    3) Ensure that the film packet is correctly positioned before making the exposure
    4) Do not utilize the patient's finger as a film-holding device
    5) Ensure that PID/tube head is stable prior to exposure

BIBLIOGRAPHY

Eastman Kodak Company. *Successful Intraoral Radiography.* Rochester, NY: Eastman Kodak Company; 1998.

Frommer, HH, Stabulas-Savage, JJ. *Radiology for the Dental Professional,* 8th ed. St. Louis, MO: Elsevier; 2005: 146–158, 216–227, 248–250.

Haring, JI, Howerton, LJ. *Dental Radiography. Principles and Techniques,* 3rd ed. St. Louis, MO: Elsevier; 2006: 274–283.

Langland, OE, Langlais, RP, Preece, JW. *Principles of Dental Imaging,* 2nd ed. Baltimore, MD: Lippincott, Williams & Wilkins; 2002: 155–172.

1. The ability to recognize errors made when taking dental radiographs will help the oral health care professional to:
   - A. Keep patient radiation exposure to a minimum
   - B. Provide optimal oral health care for the patient
   - C. Properly diagnose oral conditions
   - D. Avoid retake radiographs
   - E. All of the above

2. All of the following are characteristics of a quality periapical radiograph *except* one. Which one is this *exception?*
   - A. 2 mm of alveolar bone visible beyond the apex of each tooth.
   - B. The density of the image not too light or too dark.
   - C. The interproximal spaces appear overlapped.
   - D. The image is an accurate representation of the teeth and supporting structures.
   - E. The radiograph is free of technique and/or processing errors.

3. Which of the following errors would result in a clear or blank film?
   - A. Nonexposure to x-rays
   - B. Exposing the same film twice
   - C. Extended developing time
   - D. Accidental white light exposure

4. Which of the following would result in herringbone-error?
   - A. The film packet was bent prior to exposure.
   - B. The back of the film packet faced the x-ray beam during exposure.
   - C. The lead foil was chemically processed with the film.
   - D. The film was used to expose more than one area of the oral cavity.

5. Developer contamination of the film prior to processing results in:
   - A. A black artifact
   - B. A white artifact

6. Radiographs that are too dark result from all of the following *except* one. Which one is this *exception?*
   - A. Developer solution was too hot.
   - B. Processing time was too long.
   - C. The developer chemical mix was overactive.
   - D. White light leaking into the darkroom.
   - E. The film was placed in the fixer first.

7. The apices of the mandibular molar teeth in a periapical radiograph appear to be cut off the image. Which of the following errors is the most likely cause?
   - A. Inadequate vertical angulation
   - B. Excessive vertical angulation
   - C. Inadequate horizontal angulation
   - D. Excessive horizontal angulation

8. The image of the maxillary molar teeth in a periapical radiograph appears elongated. What should you do to improve this image?
    A. Increase the vertical angulation.
    B. Decrease the vertical angulation.
    C. Increase the horizontal angulation.
    D. Decrease the horizontal angulation.

9. Incorrect horizontal angulation results in which of the following errors?
    A. Cone-cut
    B. Overlapping
    C. Reticulation
    D. Foreshortening

10. The overhead white light in the darkroom was turned on before a film was completely inserted into the automatic processor. This is the third time this month that this error has occurred. Describe the error created. Explain how and why the resulting image appears this way. What do you think is causing this error to occur so often? What corrective actions can you suggest to prevent this error from occurring?

_____

_____

_____

_____

_____

_____

_____

_____

_____

Radiographic Quality Assurance

INTRODUCTION

Dental radiographic quality increases when a carefully administered quality assurance program is in place. Ensuring the production of diagnostic quality radiographs while also minimizing radiation exposure is the definition of quality assurance. To be effective, quality assurance requires a plan of action. This plan is referred to as quality control. Quality control is the means of testing and regulating x-ray equipment and procedures used to expose, process, and store radiographic films. The benefits of quality control include improved patient care through production of quality radiographic images, decreased radiation exposure because retake radiographs are avoided, and time and monetary savings both for patient and the oral health care practice. The time spent developing and implementing a quality assurance program is worth the benefits gained.

X-ray equipment is regulated by federal, state, and local ordinances, which usually include inspections and evaluation of equipment, but the radiographer plays an important role in the daily monitoring of equipment. It may be convenient to assign equipment testing to these expert inspectors. However, the dental radiographer is ultimately responsible for the equipment at the time of use. The dental radiographer should possess a working knowledge of the equipment utilized and understand when results produced by this equipment are below standard.

The purpose of this exercise is to introduce the student to several quality control tests that the radiographer may perform. Performing the quality control tests in this exercise provides a twofold benefit. The student will gain experience in evaluating the performance of processing and exposure equipment, and the results of these student activities may help fulfill the quality assurance required on the institution's equipment.

OBJECTIVES

Following completion of this lab activity, you will be able to:

1. Identify the role the radiographer plays in establishing and maintaining a quality assurance program.

2. Perform quality control tests on the equipment used to process dental radiographs.

3. Perform quality control tests to monitor stored dental radiographic film.

4. Perform quality control tests on the equipment used to expose dental radiographs.

5. Value establishing a quality assurance program for the oral health care practice.

MATERIALS

Size #2 radiographic films

Sample pre-fogged film

Step-wedge (commercially made or made from discarded lead foils using Procedure 9.1)

Coin (penny, nickel, dime, etc.)

Three different metal identification items (paper clip, tack, safety pin, etc.)

Viewbox

PREPARATION

1. Study the chapter outline to prepare for this laboratory exercise. An understanding of the material presented in the outline is required to complete this activity.

2. Designate an area, countertop, or operatory chair for this exercise.

3. Instructor demonstration may enhance knowledge of the laboratory exercise.

LABORATORY EXERCISE ACTIVITIES

Part 1: Quality Control Test for Effectiveness of Processing Chemistry—Reference Film

The purpose of this activity is to monitor the daily strength of the processing chemistry. Manufacturers recommend replenishing and completely changing processing solutions at preset intervals, but actual usage may dictate that solutions be changed more or less frequently than these recommendations. Ideally, solutions should be tested for optimal processing strength daily, or twice daily in the case of extremely high usage as occurs in a clinical setting. Solutions should be changed prior to reducing the quality of a patient's radiographs.

1. Obtain two size #2 radiographic film packets.

2. Check posted exposure settings for the dental x-ray unit and set for the maxillary central incisor periapical radiograph.

3. Prepare to expose the first film by placing it tube side up on the counter-top or operatory chair.

4. Place the step-wedge on top of the film packet.

5. Direct the PID over the film packet and step-wedge. Maintain a distance of 1″ between the edge of the PID and the film packet and step-wedge. (See Figure 9.3.)

6. Expose the first film and step-wedge.

7. Immediately expose the second film and step-wedge using the same x-ray unit, at the same settings, in the same manner.

8. Assuming it is the beginning of your laboratory session and that the processing chemicals are fresh, process one of the exposed films. Set the other exposed film aside to be processed at the end of the laboratory session.

9. Continue with the rest of the exercise. At the end of the laboratory session, process the film you exposed and set aside at the beginning of the laboratory session.

Part 2: Quality Control Test for Adequacy of Darkroom Safelighting—Coin Test

The purpose of this activity is to evaluate the adequacy of the safelighting conditions in the darkroom. This test is most valuable when performed as a true simulation. Because film that has been exposed, as is the case with patient films, is more sensitive to exposure by white light, you will be pre-exposing the films before performing the coin test. Additionally, allowing your test film to remain opened on the darkroom counter for two minutes will simulate the approximate time a patient's films may be exposed to the darkroom lighting conditions when opening a full mouth series of film packets aseptically. (See Laboratory Exercise 6, Infection Control and Student Partner Practice.)

1. Obtain one size #2 radiographic film packet.

2. Check posted exposure settings for the dental x-ray unit, and set at the lowest possible setting to pre-expose the film.

3. Prepare to expose the film by placing it tube side up on the counter-top or operatory chair.

4. Direct the PID over the film packet. The goal is to only slightly expose the film, so maintain a distance of 12″ between the edge of the PID and the film packet.

5. Expose the film at this low exposure setting and 12″ distance.

6. In the darkroom, secure the door, turn off the overhead white light, and turn on the safelight.

7. Open the pre-exposed film packet and place the film on a paper towel on the counter where patient films will be handled.

8. Place a coin on top of the film.

9. Wait approximately 2 minutes.

10. Remove the coin from the film.

11. Process the film as usual.

Part 3: Quality Control Test for Film Care—Fogged Film Test

The purpose of this activity is to evaluate the condition of film. Whenever a new box of film is opened, it should be tested prior to use. Use a sample prefogged film from your instructor. If a sample of fogged film is not available, you may create a fogged film to use for this exercise.

1. Obtain two size #2 radiographic film packets.

2. Check posted exposure factors for the dental x-ray unit, and set at the lowest possible setting to fog the film.

3. Prepare to fog one of the films by placing it tube side up on the countertop or operatory chair.

4. Direct the PID over the film packet. Maintain a distance of approximately 12″ between the edge of the PID and the film packet.

5. Expose the film at this low exposure setting and 12″ distance.

6. Do not expose the second film. Do not allow the second film to come in contact with stray radiation, heat, humidity, or chemical fumes.

7. In the darkroom, secure the door, turn off the overhead white light, and turn on the safelight.

8. Process both films.

Part 4: Quality Control Test for Dental X-Ray Equipment—Beam Alignment Test

The purpose of this activity is to determine the size and alignment of the primary beam. Use three different metal items to label the films during exposure. Use the beam alignment template that follows to align films for exposure and again after processing to aid in re-orienting the films.

1. Obtain four size #2 radiographic film packets.

2. Check posted exposure settings for the dental x-ray unit, and set for the maxillary central incisor periapical radiograph.

3. Place the beam alignment template on the countertop or chair designated for this activity.

4. Prepare to expose all four films by placing them tube side up on the beam alignment template on the countertop or operatory chair.

5. See the beam alignment template to line up the embossed dots on each film packet. This arrangement will help you identify the radiographs after processing.

6. Place one each of the metal identification objects on three of the films. Record which object you used on the appropriate line on the beam alignment template. The images of these objects will further help you identify where to place the films after processing.

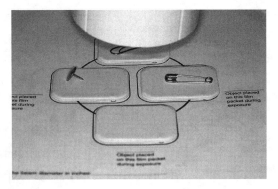

Figure 11.1 Four size #2 film packets will be placed on the beam alignment diagram to test the beam alignment. Note the arrangement of the metal objects to help identify the films after processing.

7. Direct the PID over the center of the beam alignment template. Use the template as your guide to PID placement. Approximately one-half of each of the four films will be in the path of the primary beam. Maintain a distance of 1″ between the edge of the PID and the films placed on the beam alignment diagram. (See Figure 11.1 ■.)

8. Expose the films.

9. Process the four films as usual.

Part 5: Quality Control Test for Dental X-Ray Equipment—Unit Output Test

The purpose of this activity is to evaluate the dental x-ray unit for consistency of radiation output.

1. Obtain three size #2 radiographic film packets.

2. Check posted exposure settings for the dental x-ray unit, and set for the maxillary central incisor periapical radiograph.

3. Prepare to expose the first film by placing it tube side up on the countertop or operatory chair.

4. Place a step-wedge on top of the film packet.

5. Direct the PID over the film packet and step-wedge. Maintain a distance of 1″ between the edge of the PID and the film packet-step wedge.

6. Expose the first film and step-wedge.

7. Set this exposed film aside.

8. Wait approximately **10 MINUTES.**

9. Expose the second film *in the same manner, using the same x-ray unit, at the same settings.*

10. Set this second exposed film aside.

11. Wait an additional **10 MINUTES.**

12. Expose the third film *in the same manner, using the same x-ray unit, at the same settings.*

13. Immediately process all three of the exposed films.

Part 6: Quality Control Test for X-Ray Equipment— mA Calibration

The purpose of this activity is to evaluate the radiation output as controlled by the milliamperage (mA) setting. The x-ray unit must have an adjustable mA to be able to perform this test.

1. Obtain two size #2 radiographic film packets.

2. Set the exposure settings to: **15 mA, 12 IMPULSES, at 70 kVp.**

3. Prepare to expose the first film by placing it tube side up on the countertop or operatory chair.

4. Place the step-wedge on top of the film packet.

5. Direct the PID over the film packet and step-wedge. Maintain a distance of 1″ between the edge of the PID and the film packet step-wedge.

6. Expose the first film and step-wedge.

7. Set this exposed film aside.

8. Change the exposure settings to: **10 mA, 18 IMPULSES, at 70 kVp.**

9. Prepare to expose the second film by placing it tube side up on the countertop or operatory chair.

10. Place the step-wedge on top of the film packet.

11. Direct the PID over the film packet and step-wedge. Maintain a distance of 1″ between the edge of the PID and the film packet and step-wedge.

12. Expose the second film and step-wedge.

13. Process the two films as usual.

COMPETENCY AND EVALUATION

1. Mount the processed films on the simulated film mounts that follow. Secure with a piece of tape placed along the top edge of the film only, so that the films may be raised slightly to allow light underneath for ease of viewing.

   NOTE: **USE THE LABIAL MOUNTING METHOD. THE RAISED PORTION OF THE EMBOSSED DOT IS TOWARD YOU (CONVEX) WHEN PLACING THE FILM ONTO THE PAGE.**

2. Place the page with the mounted films taped to it on a view box and evaluate. Examine the results of the quality control tests performed in each of the six parts of this exercise. Based on your results, summarize the following in your own words:

   a. Referring to the quality control test performed in Part 1 of this exercise, what is your assessment of the processing chemistry? Why?

b. Referring to the quality control test performed in Part 2 of this exercise, what is your assessment of the darkroom safe-lighting? Why?

c. Referring to the quality control test performed in Part 3 of this exercise, how can you tell that a film is fogged? What effect will film fogging have on the quality of the radiograph?

d. Referring to the quality control test performed in Part 4 of this exercise, what is your assessment of the x-ray beam of the dental x-ray unit you tested? Why?

e. Referring to the quality control test performed in Part 5 of this exercise, what is your assessment of the radiation output of the machine you tested? Why?

f. Referring to the quality control test performed in Part 6 of this exercise, what is your assessment of the milliamperage setting on the dental x-ray unit you tested? Why?

3. Complete the study questions.

Beam Alignment Template

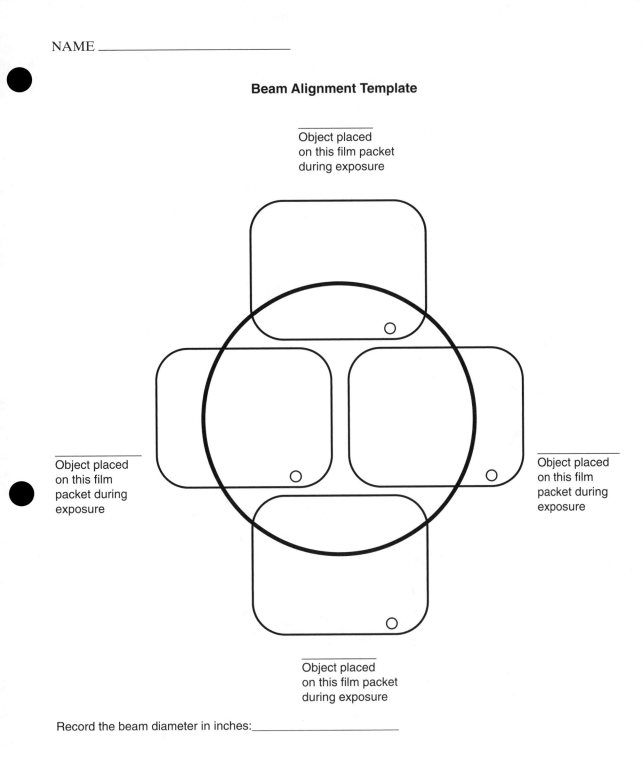

_____
Object placed
on this film packet
during exposure

_____
Object placed
on this film
packet during
exposure

_____
Object placed
on this film
packet during
exposure

_____
Object placed
on this film packet
during exposure

Record the beam diameter in inches:_____

NAME _____

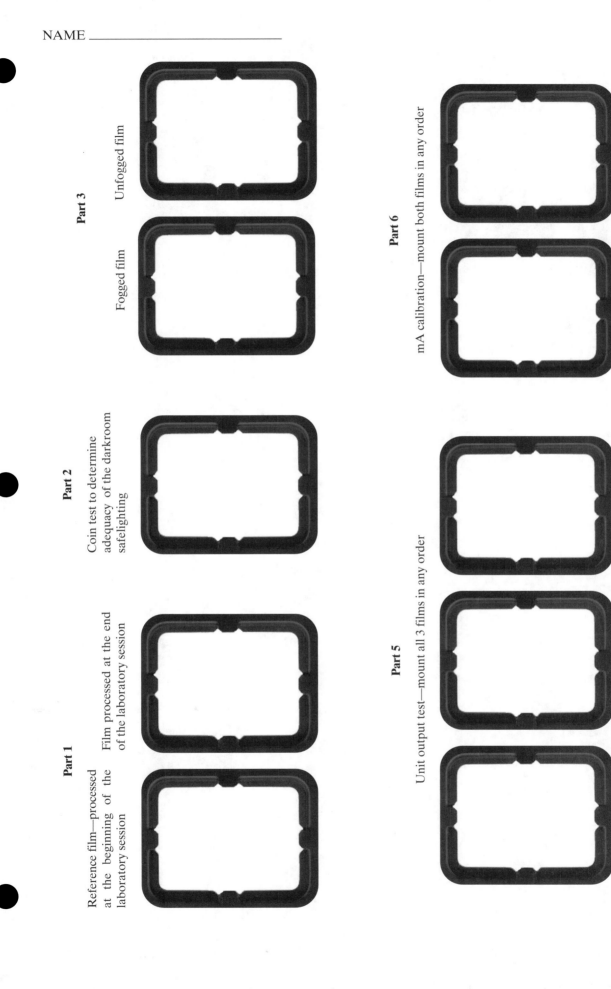

Part 1

Reference film—processed at the beginning of the laboratory session

Film processed at the end of the laboratory session

Part 2

Coin test to determine adequacy of the darkroom safelighting

Part 3

Fogged film

Unfogged film

Part 5

Unit output test—mount all 3 films in any order

Part 6

mA calibration—mount both films in any order

I. Quality assurance
    A. Producing diagnostic quality radiographs while minimizing patient radiation exposure
    B. Quality administration
        1. Responsibility includes the entire oral health care team
            a. Dentist
            b. Dental hygienist
            c. Dental assistant
            d. Qualified expert technician—as required by law
        2. Guidelines for developing and maintaining a quality assurance program
            a. Assess quality assurance needs
            b. Develop quality assurance plan
            c. Assign authority
            d. Provide training
            e. Maintain schedule
            f. Document actions
            g. Evaluate quality assurance plan
    C. Quality control
        1. Specific tests to evaluate quality assurance
            a. Dental x-ray equipment assessment
                1) X-ray unit output test
                    a) Measures the amount of radiation at standard settings over time.
                    b) Utilizes a dosimeter to record output and compare for consistency.
                    c) May also be evaluated with a step-wedge.
                    d) Films exposed at standard settings over time with a step-wedge can be compared for consistency in density.
                    e) Failed test requires attention by qualified expert technician.
                2) Exposure timer test
                    a) Measures accuracy of the impulse timer.
                    b) Utilizes a commercially made brass spinning top.
                    c) Set the top in motion on an intraoral film packet (Figure 11.2 ■).

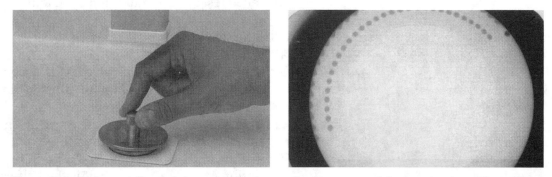

Figure 11.2 Commercially made brass top used to evaluate accuracy of the impulse timer. The radiolucent "dots" on the processed film should equal the number of impulses set. (Reprinted courtesy of Eastman Kodak Company. *Quality Control Tests for Dental Radiography.* Rochester, NY: 1994.)

    d) Expose the film packet with the top spinning.

    e) After processing, count the radiolucent "dots" indicating exposure through the holes in the spinning top to verify accuracy of the timer.

    f) Failed test requires attention by qualified expert technician.

3) Milliamperage setting test

    a) Measures accuracy of the mA dial.

    b) Utilizes a step-wedge.

    c) Expose the step-wedge to varied mA and impulse settings while maintaining constant milliamperage-impulses (or milliamperage-seconds).

      (1) For example:

$$10 \text{ mA} \times 18 \text{ impulses} = 180 \text{ mAi}$$
$$15 \text{ mA} \times 12 \text{ impulses} = 180 \text{ mAi}$$

      (2) For example:

$$10 \text{ mA} \times 0.3 \text{ seconds} = 3 \text{ mAs}$$
$$15 \text{ mA} \times 0.2 \text{ seconds} = 3 \text{ mAs}$$

    d) Films exposed to the same mAi product should appear similar in density.

    e) Failed test requires attention by qualified expert technician.

4) Kilovoltage setting test

    a) Measures accuracy of the kVp dial.

    b) Utilizes a commercially made kilovoltage measuring instrument to calibrate the dial setting with actual kVp output.

    c) Failed test requires attention by qualified expert technician.

5) Focal spot size test

    a) Measures the image unsharpness created by an enlarged focal spot area. Over time, bombarding electrons can cause pitting and therefore enlargement of the focal spot area.

    b) Utilizes a commercially made focal spot test tool to measure the image unsharpness produced by the focal spot.

    c) Failed test requires attention by qualified expert technician.

6) Filtration test

    a) Measures the penetrating power of the x-ray beam.

    b) Utilizes the test for half value layer which places commercially available aluminum filters of varying thicknesses in the path of the beam.

    c) A dosimeter is required to measure the amount of radiation able to penetrate the filters.

    d) The thickness of the filter required to reduce the radiation exposure by one-half is the half value layer.

    e) Failed test requires attention by qualified expert technician.

7) Beam collimation test
   a) Evaluates the beam diameter and alignment.
   b) Utilizes four size #2 intraoral films, or one size #4 intraoral film, or an extraoral film loaded into a cassette with intensifying screens.
   c) Direct the PID over the film(s) and expose.
   d) Evaluate the image for size (beam diameter must be no greater than 2.75″ (7 cm) and edge definition (sharpness).
   e) Failed test requires an inspection of the lead collimator at the base of the PID to ensure that it is seated properly; also the PID should be properly seated into the tube head opening.
8) Tube head drift assessment (Figure 11.3 ■)
   a) Evaluates the stability of the tube head in various positions.
   b) Extend the support arm and place the tube head in the various positions required to expose all areas of the oral cavity; observe for drift and/or change of position.
   c) Failed test requires that the support arm be adjusted according to the manufacturer's instructions to eliminate drift and/or vibration.
b. Dental x-ray film processing equipment
   1) Darkroom adequacy assessment
      a) Evaluates for white light leak.
      b) Utilizes a visual inspection.
         (1) Enter the darkroom, turn off all lights, including white overhead light and safelighting.
         (2) Allow eyes to become accustomed to the dark, and then visually scan the room for white light leaks.
         (3) Check, for example, around doors, pipes, ventilation ducts, and so on.
         (4) Use chalk if necessary to mark area of white light leak for location later when white light is turned on.
         (5) Inspect darkroom for any other light sources that are not red (safe) in color, such as luminous indicator dials on equipment, luminous wristwatch faces, and so on.

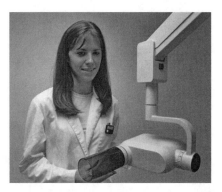

Figure 11.3 Radiographer evaluating the stability of the tube head in various positions.

c) Failed test requires applying a mask or block to the white light leak.

2) Safelight test
   a) Evaluates the safelight for film fog.
   b) Utilizes the coin test.
      (1) Preexpose an intraoral film to sensitize the crystals within the emulsion.
      (2) Unwrap the film under safelight conditions.
      (3) Place unwrapped film on the darkroom counter, place coin on top of the film to shield this portion of the film from all light in the room. (Figure 11.4 ■)
      (4) Allow the film to remain on the counter under these conditions for approximately 2 minutes.
      (5) Process the film and evaluate for an image of the coin indicating unsafe lighting. (Figure 11.5 ■)
   c) Failed test requires an inspection of the condition of the safelight filter, evaluating for scratches, proper seal; also evaluate the filter color (red is appropriate for all dental x-ray film types), bulb wattage (15 watts or less is considered safe for all types of dental x-ray films), distance away from the working area (a minimum of 4′ above the counter is considered safe for all types of dental x-ray films).

3) Processing chemistry test
   a) Evaluates the efficacy of processing chemistry
   b) Utilizes a reference film
      (1) Expose several intraoral films (the number of films exposed depends on the usage load on the processing chemistry—30 exposed films may be needed for those practices whose chemistry will probably require changing in 30 days; seven films may be adequate for those practices in which chemistry is changed weekly). Use a step-wedge, and expose the films with the same unit at the same settings.
      (2) Process one of the exposed films in new chemistry, store the remaining films in a safe place (away from radiation, heat, humidity, chemical fumes).
      (3) Attach the processed film with the step-wedge image to a view box. At the beginning of each day,

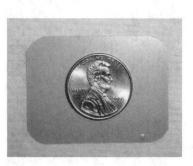

Figure 11.4 Coin test for determining adequacy of the safelight conditions in the darkroom.

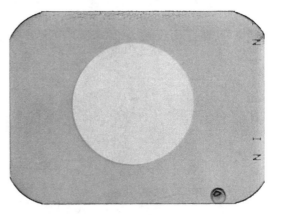

Figure 11.5 Coin test results indicating unsafe light conditions. Note the outline of the coin.

obtain one of the exposed films and process normally; compare each subsequent film to the reference film. The density of each film should match the density observed in the reference film.

    c) Failed test is indicated when the newly processed film image of the step-wedge appears lighter than the reference film; the processing solutions should be replaced with fresh chemicals.

c. Dental x-ray film assessment
  1) Proper film storage test
    a) Evaluates the condition of dental x-ray film.
    b) Utilizes one film from a freshly opened new box.
    c) Open the film under safelight conditions and process normally.
    d) Inspect the processed film for fog.
    e) Failed test requires checking the expiration date on the film box. Use oldest film first to assist in using film prior to expiration date; evaluate the film storage area for possible fogging from radiation, excess heat and/or humidity, chemical fumes.

d. Dental radiograph viewing conditions assessment
  1) View box inspection
    a) Evaluates the condition of the view box to enhance interpretation and diagnosis.
    b) Utilizes visual inspection to assess the view box for fluorescent bulb flicker or a color change to black indicating bulb failure.
    c) Visually inspect view box surface for scratches and debris.
    d) Failed inspection requires replacing the bulb and/or cleaning the view box surface.

e. Extraoral dental radiographic assessment
  1) Film cassette inspection
    a) Assess the condition of the cassette to prevent film fog due to light leaking into the cassette and to ensure a tight contact between film and intensifying screens.

b) Utilize a visual inspection to examine the lock/snap mechanism for securing the cassette. (Figure 11.6 ■)
c) Utilize a commercial product called a wire mesh test object to evaluate the film/intensifying screen contact.
(1) Expose the wire mesh test object, and process the extraoral film as usual.
(2) View the image of the wire mesh test object for good film/intensifying screen contact.
d) Failed assessment requires repairing or replacing the damaged cassette.
2) Intensifying screens inspection
a) Evaluate the condition of the intensifying screens to avoid the presence of artifacts, which hinder interpretation and diagnosis.
b) Utilize a visual inspection of intensifying screens. Look for scratches, debris, or worn areas.
c) Failed test requires cleaning or replacement of the intensifying screens. Avoid over-cleaning intensifying screens; clean only as needed.

II. Documentation
A. Post instructions
1. Dental x-ray unit recommended settings should be posted near the control panel to eliminate exposure errors.
2. Processing instructions should be posted in the darkroom to eliminate processing errors.
3. Other procedures such as extraoral radiographic exposures, film duplicating, and film identification methods should have posted instructions.
B. Maintenance schedule log
1. Record when each quality control test is due and performed, and document the results and corrective action taken (if it was necessary).
2. Assign maintenance duties and authority.
C. Maintain an error log
1. Identify retake errors and corrective action taken, and record in writing.

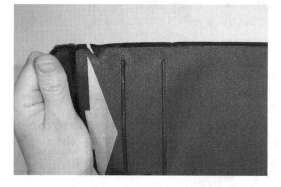

Figure 11.6 Visual inspection of this cassette reveals tears that may be allowing white light to enter the cassette and expose the film.

2. Use this log as a basis for identifying areas that need preventive quality control action.
3. Use this log as a basis for in-service and retraining personnel.

BIBLIOGRAPHY

Eastman Kodak Company: *Quality Assurance in Dental Film Radiography.* Available at www.kodak.com/global/plugins/acrobat/en/health/pdf/prod/dental/N-416.pdf. Accessed April 27, 2006.

Eastman Kodak Company. *Quality Control Tests for Dental Radiography.* Rochester, NY: Eastman Kodak Company; 1997.

Eastman Kodak Company: *Exposure and Processing for Dental Film Radiography.* Available at www.kodak.com/global/plugins/acrobat/en/health/pdf/prod/dental/N-413.pdf. Accessed April 27, 2006.

Haring, JI, Howerton, LJ. *Dental Radiography. Principles and Techniques,* 3rd ed. St. Louis, MO: Elsevier; 2006: 128–136.

Langlais, RP. *Kodak Dental Radiograph Series: Extra Oral Radiography.* Rochester, NY: Eastman Kodak Company; 1989.

Langland, OE, Langlais, RP, Preece, JW. *Principles of Dental Imaging,* 2nd ed. Baltimore, MD: Lippincott Williams & Wilkins; 2002: 179–192.

Lusk, LT. Peak performance. *RDH.* 1997: 3:32, 37–38.

1. Who is responsible for administration of a quality assurance program?
   A. Dentist
   B. Dental hygienist
   C. Dental assistant
   D. All of the above

2. All of the following are quality control tests for the dental x-ray unit *except* one. Which one is this *exception?*
   A. Unit output
   B. Beam alignment
   C. Tube head stability
   D. TLD badge evaluation

3. A step-wedge can be used to test all of the following *except* one. Which one is this *exception?*
   A. X-ray unit output
   B. Exposure timer
   C. mA setting
   D. Processing chemistry

4. A commercially made brass top is used to evaluate the accuracy of the
   A. kVp setting
   B. mA setting
   C. impulse timer
   D. filtration

5. Placing aluminium filters of varying thickness in the path of the x-ray beam tests the
   A. safelight
   B. step-wedge
   C. half-value layer
   D. beam collimation

6. Which of the following beam diameters is within acceptable limits?
   A. 2.75″
   B. 3.75″
   C. 4.75″
   D. 5.75″

7. The coin test may be used to determine which of the following?
   A. Film density
   B. Processing errors
   C. Safelight adequacy
   D. Unit output

8. The outline of the coin imaged onto the film as a result of the coin test would indicate?
   A. A successful test
   B. A failed test

9. A reference film is a radiograph processed under ideal conditions, *and* then used to monitor the efficacy of the processing chemistry.

    A. The first part of the statement is true, the second part of the statement is false.

    B. The first part of the statement is false, the second part of the statement is true.

    C. Both parts of the statement are true and related.

    D. Both parts of the statement are true, but not related.

    E. Both parts of the statement are false.

10. All of the following play a role in the inspection of extraoral radiography intensifying screens *except* one. Which one is this *exception?*

    A. Perform a visual inspection for scratches.

    B. Check to remove debris periodically.

    C. Clean with appropriate cleanser after every use.

    D. Utilize the wire mesh test object to check for film-screen contact.

Radiographic Interpretation

INTRODUCTION

Dental hygienists and dental assistants play an important role in radiographic interpretation. Although it is the dentist's responsibility for the final diagnosis and treatment of oral lesions, all members of the oral health care team should be able to recognize radiographic deviations from the normal. Patient care is only enhanced when radiographs are interpreted, and findings that deviate from normal radiographic anatomy are called to the attention of the dentist. The ability to read and explain radiographic findings to the patient is an important skill performed by the radiographer.

Furthermore, developing interpretation skills fosters an appreciation for obtaining quality radiographs. Knowing what information is being sought from a radiographic image motivates the radiographer to obtain precise images. For example, a slight film packet placement error may at first seem insignificant. However, when film packet placement is accurate and disease is revealed that would not have been diagnosed from the incorrectly placed film, the radiographer begins to understand the importance of radiographic skills. (Figure 12.1 ■)

Interpretation is a skill that requires practice. The beginner may easily become frustrated by a seeming inability to see what the expert easily identifies. Furthermore, because radiographs are two-dimensional representations of three-dimensional structures, image variations of normal anatomical landmarks may confuse the beginner interpreter. Varying radiographic density may also alter the appearance of normal anatomy. For these reasons, it is important to understand that the basis for developing interpretative skills is a solid working knowledge of normal radiographic anatomy. When interpreting a radiographic image, the radiographer should

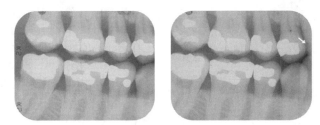

Figure 12.1 The premolar bitewing radiograph on the left was not positioned to image the distal portion of the maxillary canine. When correctly positioned to image the distal portion of the canine, as in the film on the right, the carious lesion is clearly visible.

first identify normal anatomy, then systematically progress through a sequence of evaluation, assigning a name to every radiopacity and radiolucency observed.

For the purpose of organizing the learning process, this exercise divides the interpretative practice into five categories: (1) tooth development and anomalies, (2) dental materials, (3) periodontal disease, (4) caries, and (5) other common oral conditions. By organizing the interpretation process in this manner, the student is less likely to omit or not see something that should have been identified on the radiograph. The student will be prompted, through the use of radiographic interpretation forms, to evaluate radiographic images systematically. The purpose of this exercise is to provide the student with structured, systematic practice at learning how to interpret dental radiographs in these five areas. Prior to beginning this exercise, the student should possess a working knowledge of dental materials, normal anatomy, and oral conditions that deviate from normal before attempting to identify these radiographically.

OBJECTIVES

Following completion of this lab activity, you will be able to:

1. Identify tooth development and common anomalies radiographically.

2. Identify common dental materials radiographically.

3. Identify periodontal bone loss radiographically.

4. Identify caries radiographically.

MATERIALS

Viewbox

Magnifying device

Periodontal probe

Sample patient radiographs

PREPARATION

1. Study the chapter outline to prepare for this laboratory exercise. An understanding of the material presented in the outline is required to complete this activity.

2. Designate an area with a viewbox and countertop for this exercise.

3. View the radiographs that accompany each of the 4 parts of this exercise.

4. Using the Radiographic Interpretation Form appropriate for each of the 4 parts, document your interpretion of the radiographs. Note that not all conditions are present on the sample radiographs provided. Nevertheless, it is important that radiographs be examined for the presence of all possible conditions.

5. Your instructor may provide you with additional sample radiographs. The Radiographic Interpretation Forms may be copied and used to

interpret the patient radiographs available from your instructor for additional practice or you may be directed to use the interpretation form available at your facility.

LABORATORY EXERCISE ACTIVITIES

Part 1: Interpretation—Tooth Development and Abnormalities

View the radiographs and using the Radiographic Interpretation Form—Tooth Development and Abnormalities record findings.

Part 2: Interpretation—Dental Materials

View the radiographs and using the Radiographic Interpretation Form—Dental Materials record findings.

Part 3: Interpretation—Periodontal Disease

View the radiographs and using the Radiographic Interpretation Form—Periodontal Disease record findings.

Part 4: Interpretation—Caries

View the radiographs and using the Radiographic Interpretation Form—Caries record findings.

COMPETENCY AND EVALUATION

1. Did using a form help you proceed through the interpretive process? In what ways did the simulated forms presented here, or the form your instructor gave you, guide you through the interpretive process?

2. Compare your completed forms with other students in the class. Did you identify the same conditions or do your interpretations differ? In what ways?

3. Complete the study questions.

Part 1: Tooth Development and Anomalies

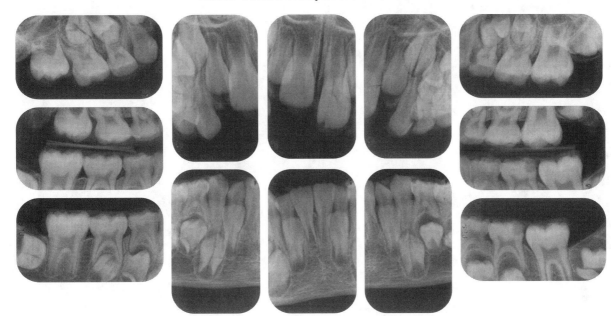

Radiographic Interpretation Form—Tooth Development and Anomalies

View the radiographs for evidence of the conditions listed in the column at the right. View tooth #1 (maxillary right third molar) and vicinity. Begin the interpretation process in the maxillary right. View tooth #1 (maxillary right third molar) and vicinity. If tooth #1 is not present radiographically, "X" out the tooth number and begin the interpretation process with tooth #2 (maxillary right second molar). If tooth #1 is present radiographically, circle the tooth number and then proceed to evaluate tooth #1 for the conditions listed in the column on the right. Evaluate both permanent and primary teeth and vicinity for these conditions.

Condition present:

Tooth # 1 2 3 4 5 6 7 8 9 10 11 12 13 14 15 16 17 18 19 20 21 22 23 24 25 26 27 28 29 30 31 32

- Unerupted/impacted
- Congenitally missing/supernumerary
- Fusion/gemination
- Taurodontia/pulp stones
- Root dilaceration/supernumerary root
- Dens en dente/enamel pearl
- Macrodontia/microdontia
- External resorption/internal resorption

Tooth # A B C D E F G H I J K L M N O P Q R S T

- Unerupted/impacted
- Congenitally missing/supernumerary
- Fusion/gemination
- Taurodontia/pulp stones
- Root dilaceration/supernumerary root
- Dens en dente/enamel pearl
- Macrodontia/microdontia
- External resorption/internal resorption
- Other

Part 2: Dental Materials

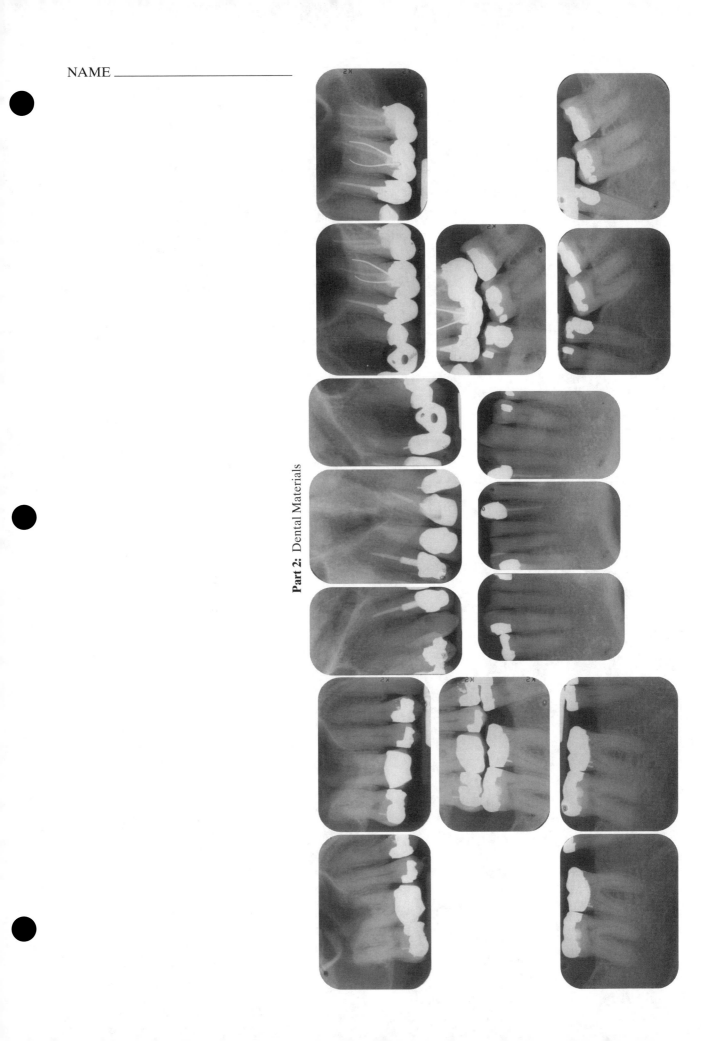

Radiographic Interpretation Form—Dental Materials

View the radiographs for the presence of these restorative materials. Begin the interpretation process in the maxillary right. View tooth #1 (maxillary right third molar). If tooth #1 is not present radiographically, "X" out the tooth number and begin the interpretation process with tooth #2 (maxillary right second molar). If tooth #1 is present radiographically, circle the tooth number and then proceed to evaluate tooth #1 for the presence of any of the materials listed in the column on the right. Check all materials present. (For example, tooth #1 may have a metallic crown, endodontic filling and also be an abutment.)

Dental materials present:

Tooth #	Metallic restoration (amalgam)	Metallic crown (gold, semi-precious metal)	Stainless steel crown	Porcelain fused to metal crown	Porcelain crown (porcelain jacket, veneer)	Composite restoration (silicate, acrylic)	Temporary restoration	Sealant	Base material	Cement	Retention pin	Post and core	Endodontic filling (gutta percha, silver points)	Implant	Orthodontic appliance	Abutment	Pontic	Other (foreign object such as amalgam tatoo, facial jewelry, etc.)
1																		
2																		
3																		
4																		
5																		
6																		
7																		
8																		
9																		
10																		
11																		
12																		
13																		
14																		
15																		
16																		
17																		
18																		
19																		
20																		
21																		
22																		
23																		
24																		
25																		
26																		
27																		
28																		
29																		
30																		
31																		
32																		

Part 3: Periodontal Disease

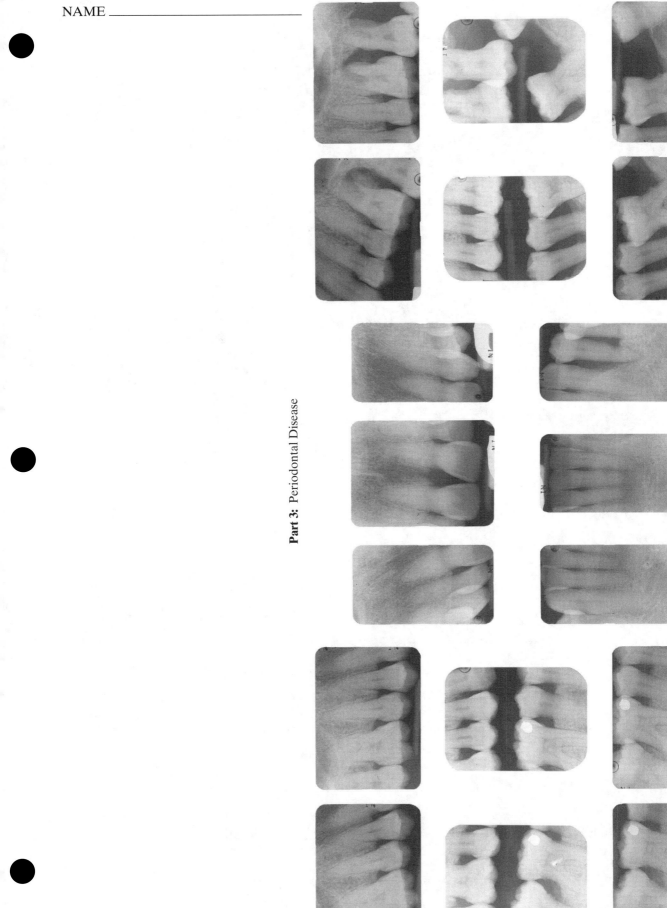

NAME _____

Radiographic Interpretation Form—Periodontal Disease

View the radiographs for evidence of periodontal disease and predisposing factors. Begin the interpretation process in the maxillary right. View tooth #1 (maxillary right third molar). If tooth #1 is not present radiographically, "X" out the tooth number and begin the interpretation process with tooth #2 (maxillary right second molar). If tooth #1 is present radiographically, circle the tooth number and then proceed to evaluate tooth #1 for evidence of any of the conditions listed in the column on the right. Check all conditions present. (For example, tooth #1 may have a calculus present, bone loss, and furcation involvement.)

Tooth #

Periodontal condition present:

Tooth #	1	2	3	4	5	6	7	8	9	10	11	12	13	14	15	16	17	18	19	20	21	22	23	24	25	26	27	28	29	30	31	32	Periodontal condition present:
																																	Calculus
																																	Overhanging or defective restoration or poorly contoured crown margins
																																	Open contact
																																	Widening of PDL space
																																	Triangulation
																																	Early bone loss (indistinct lamina dura, fuzzy radiolucency in crestal bone area)
																																	Moderate bone loss (distinct cupping out of the crestal bone, 30–50% loss compared to length of tooth root)
																																	Advanced bone loss (crestal bone loss is >50% compared to length of tooth root)
																																	Horizontal bone loss
																																	Vertical bone loss
																																	Furcation involvement
																																	Evidence of tooth mobility (drift)
																																	Periodontal abscess
																																	Other (specify)

Part 4: Caries

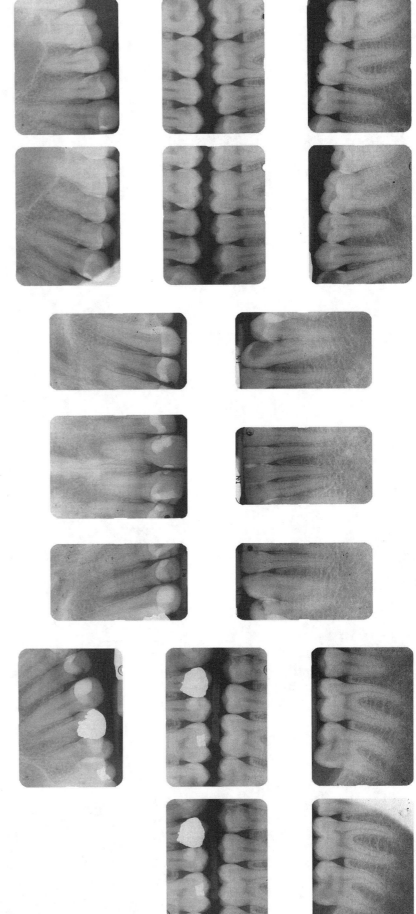

Radiographic Interpretation Form—Caries

View the radiographs for evidence of caries and defective restorations. Begin the interpretation process in the maxillary right. View tooth #1 (maxillary right third molar). If tooth #1 is not present radiographically, "X" out the tooth number and begin the interpretation process with tooth #2 (maxillary right second molar). If tooth #1 is present radiographically, circle the tooth number and then proceed to evaluate tooth #1 for evidence of any of the conditions listed in the column on the right. Remember that cervical burnout, abrasion, attrition, and erosion may all mimic decay. Do not record these conditions, and do not confuse them with caries.

Caries present:

Tooth #	1	2	3	4	5	6	7	8	9	10	11	12	13	14	15	16	17	18	19	20	21	22	23	24	25	26	27	28	29	30	31	32
Mesial surface caries (incipient - <1/2 through the enamel toward the DEJ)																																
Mesial surface caries (moderate - >1/2 through the enamel, but does not yet involve the DEJ)																																
Mesial surface caries (advanced - extends through the DEJ, but <1/2 way toward the pulp)																																
Mesial surface caries (severe - extends through the DEJ and >1/2 way toward the pulp)																																
Distal surface caries (incipient - <1/2 through the enamel toward the DEJ)																																
Distal surface caries (moderate - >1/2 through the enamel, but does not yet involve the DEJ)																																
Distal surface caries (advanced - extends through the DEJ, but <1/2 way toward the pulp)																																
Distal surface caries (severe - extends through the DEJ and >1/2 way toward the pulp)																																
Occlusal caries (moderate - thin radiolucent line apical to the occlusal enamel)																																
Occlusal caries (severe - radiolucency extending toward the pulp, crown missing or fractured)																																
Buccal or lingual caries																																
Root caries																																
Recurrent decay																																
Overhanging or defective restoration or poorly contoured crown margins																																
Other (specify)																																

I. Radiographic interpretation
  A. Interpretation skills are required by the
    1. Dental assistant
    2. Dental hygienist
    3. Dentist
  B. Requirements
    1. Thorough knowledge of normal radiographic anatomy
    2. Quality radiographs
    3. Mounted films
      a. Provide systematic viewing
      b. Opaque mounts block extraneous light to aid viewing
    4. Light source
      a. Viewbox
      b. Subdued room lighting
    5. Magnification
    6. Probe or other measuring device
  C. Systematic viewing
    1. Examine the entire radiograph.
    2. Begin the examination on the maxillary right side, proceed to the maxillary left, then to the mandibular left, and finish examination on the mandibular right.
    3. Use adjacent radiographs to compare views.
    4. Use a chart or diagram to record each of the following:
      a. Presence or absence of teeth
      b. Anomalies such as impactions, unerupted or transposed teeth, congenitally missing teeth
      c. Dental materials
      d. Periodontal disease
        1) Note alveolar bone height.
        2) Identify local irritating factors such as calculus and overhanging restorations.
        3) Examine the periodontal ligament space, document widening, triangulation.
      e. Caries
        1) View all surfaces of each tooth.
        2) Examine the contact point for proximal decay.
        3) Examine restoration margins for recurrent decay.
        4) Examine the area just apical to the enamel for occlusal decay.
        5) Examine for buccal/lingual decay.
      f. Oral pathology
        1) Identify and examine every anatomic structure visible on the film; assign a name to each radiopacity and radiolucency; note when some part of the image cannot be identified.
        2) Examine the bone around each tooth, noting density and trabecular pattern, compare with views in adjacent films and compare left and right sides for symmetry.

3) Examine the periodontal ligament space, observing asymmetry or breaks in the continuity.
4) Examine the pulp chamber of each tooth.
5. Record substantive radiographic deviations from the norm, documenting location, size, shape, borders, symmetry, and density.
6. Use a probe or other measuring device to document size.
7. Use previous radiographs for comparison.
   a. Compare to previous radiographs only after a thorough evaluation of the current radiographs.
   b. Do not allow previous radiographs to influence or prejudice the initial interpretation of the current radiographs.

II. Radiographic appearance of tooth development and anomalies
  A. Advantages of the use of radiographs in evaluating tooth development and detecting anomalies
    1. Assess growth and development
    2. Asymptomatic abnormalities detected
    3. Documentation of the patient's condition at a specific point in time
  B. Limitations of the use of radiographs in evaluating tooth development and detecting anomalies
    1. Radiographic findings should be utilized in conjunction with the clinical examination.
    2. Two-dimensional radiographs of three-dimensional structures may miss or mimic a developmental anomaly.
  C. Tooth development
    1. Circular radiolucent dental sac.
    2. Enamel cusps first to calcify and appear radiopaque.
    3. Crown develops as a radiopacity surrounded by a radiolucent follicle.
    4. Crown erupts as roots continue to form.
    5. Roots first appear open, dental papilla.
       a. Dental papilla should not be confused with periapical pathology.
       b. Differentiate from a periapical lesion by the age of the patient and stage of tooth development and by the presence of a contributing condition such as a large carious lesion.
    6. Root apices close, completing tooth development.
  D. Tooth eruption patterns
    1. Various stages of tooth development may be visible.
    2. As permanent tooth develops, causes resorption of the primary tooth roots.
    3. First, second, third permanent molars do not have primary predecessors.
    4. Supernumerary tooth.
    5. Congenitally missing tooth.
    6. Variations in tooth roots.
       a. Supernumerary roots
       b. Dilacerated roots
    7. Mal-positioned tooth.
       a. Transposed teeth

E. Anomalies
   1. Macrodontia
      a. Appears as a larger than normal tooth
      b. Differentiate from image magnification
   2. Microdontia
      a. Appears as a smaller than normal tooth
      b. More common occurrence in maxillary lateral incisors (peg laterals) and the third molars
   3. Gemination
      a. Appears as two crowns fused together sharing one root and root canal structure
      b. Differentiate from fusion by identifying the presence of the adjacent teeth
   4. Fusion
      a. Appears as two crowns and two root and root canal structures fused together
      b. Differentiate from gemination by identifying the absence of an adjacent tooth
   5. Concrescence
      a. Teeth appear joined by cementum
      b. Very difficult to diagnosis radiographically
      c. Teeth with roots in close proximity and/or the angle of the x-ray beam often mimic this anomaly
   6. Dens invaginatus
      a. Appearance of a "tooth within a tooth"
      b. Invagination of enamel within the pulp chamber
   7. Enamel pearl
      a. Appears as a radiopaque sphere attached to the tooth surface in the cervical region
      b. Differentiate from pulp stone by its location outside of the pulp chamber
   8. Taurodontism
      a. Appears as an enlarged pulp chamber, resembling a bull (tauros–bull; odont–tooth)
      b. Usually affects mandibular molar teeth
III. Radiographic appearance of dental materials
  A. Advantages of the use of radiographs in identifying and evaluating dental materials
     1. Document the condition of restoration margins.
     2. Assess past dental procedures such as endodontic therapy, apicoectomy, and extraction sites.
     3. Aid in documentation, dental charting.
  B. Limitations of the use of radiographs in identifying and evaluating dental materials
     1. Some dental materials are not readily distinguishable radiographically.
     2. Some dental materials may mimic caries.
  C. Radiopaque
     1. Amalgam
       a. Differentiate from other materials by irregular margins.

    b. May cover one or multiple surfaces of the tooth crown.

    c. Amalgam tatoo may appear as a radiopaque metal scrap outside the tooth, embedded in soft tissue.

2. Metal crown

    a. Differentiate from other materials by smooth margins.

    b. Usually covers entire tooth crown.

    c. Gold cannot be distinguished radiographically from other semiprecious metals.

    d. Stainless steel crown may appear less radiopaque with a "see through" appearance.

    e. Porcelain, which appears less radiopaque than metal, may be visible in a porcelain fused-to-metal crown.

3. Gold onlay and inlay

    a. Difficult to distinguish from other metal restorations

    b. Usually appear to have smooth, regular margins

    c. Do not usually cover the entire tooth crown

4. Composite

    a. Less radiopaque than metal restorations

    b. Radiopacity similar to dentin

5. Porcelain

    a. Less radiopaque than metal restorations.

    b. Radiopacity similar to dentin.

    c. May be used in porcelain fused-to-metal crowns, where the porcelain may be visible on the incisal/occlusal edge beyond the metal portion of the crown.

    d. When used as a single material, prepared tooth is visible beneath the porcelain crown.

6. Temporary filling material

    a. Less radiopaque than metal restorations

    b. Radiopacity similar to dentin

    c. Irregular margins help differentiate from composite

7. Base material

    a. Radiopacity similar to dentin

    b. May require close examination under the margin of large amalgam or composite restoration to detect radiographically

8. Cement

    a. Radiopacity varies, may appear as radiopaque as a metal.

    b. When visible radiographically, usually appears beneath a porcelain crown.

9. Sealant

    a. Radiopacity very similar to dentin

    b. Requires careful examination of the area just beneath the occlusal enamel to detect radiographically

10. Retention pin

    a. Differentiate from other materials by shape.

    b. Unique shape usually easily distinguishable.

    c. May require a close examination near margin of large amalgams, crowns to detect

    d. Appears embedded in the enamel only; will not perforate the pulp chamber

11. Post and core
    a. Differentiate from other materials by shape.
    b. Unique shape usually easily distinguishable.
    c. Location in pulp chamber helps distinguish this material from retention pin.
    d. If post and core present, tooth must also have had endodontic therapy.
12. Silver points
    a. Differentiate from other materials by shape and location.
    b. Located in root canals.
    c. More radiopaque than gutta percha.
13. Gutta percha
    a. Differentiate from other materials by shape and location.
    b. Located in root canals.
    c. Less radiopaque than silver points.
14. Implants
    a. Differentiate from other materials by shape and location.
    b. Located in area of missing tooth/teeth.
    c. Appears imbedded in alveolar bone.
    d. Restoration; usually crown and/or crown and bridge attached.
15. Fixed orthodontic appliances
    a. Differentiate from other materials by shape and location.
    b. Unique shape usually easily distinguishable.

D. Radiolucent
  1. Composite
    a. Older composite materials may appear radiolucent.
    b. Regular margins that appear prepared and location in the anterior teeth help differentiate composite from caries.
  2. Silicate
    a. Older silicate materials may appear radiolucent.
    b. Regular margins that appear prepared and location in the anterior teeth help differentiate silicate from caries.
  3. Acrylic
    a. Older acrylic materials may appear radiolucent.
    b. Regular margins that appear prepared and location in the anterior teeth help differentiate acrylic from caries.

IV. Radiographic appearance of periodontal disease
A. Advantages of the use of radiographs in the evaluation of periodontal health
  1. Images the condition of supporting bone
  2. Locates the presence of predisposing factors
  3. Aids in treatment planning and implementation by identifying infraboney defects, tooth morphology
  4. Aids in prognosis by imaging root-to-crown ratio
B. Limitations of the use of radiographs in the evaluation of periodontal health
  1. Radiographs do not image early changes in the periodontium.
  2. Actual destruction of periodontal tissue is more advanced than radiographically imaged.
  3. Two-dimensional image may hide infraboney defects.

4. Soft-to-hard tissue ratio not imaged.

5. Cannot distinguish between active and inactive disease status.

    C. Radiographic techniques

      1. Paralleling technique

        a. Parallel central ray of the x-ray beam images alveolar bone more accurately than bisecting technique.

        b. Bitewing radiographs, particularly vertical bitewing radiographs, easily provide an accurate representation of the alveolar bone.

        c. Periapical radiographs require precise vertical angulation to achieve the accurate representation of the alveolar bone imaged with bitewing radiographs.

      2. kVp

        a. Higher kVp setting produces a long scale (low contrast) image.

        b. Low contrast will image subtle changes in the periodontium.

    D. Local predisposing factors imaged by radiographs

      1. Calculus

      2. Overhanging restorations

      3. Occlusal trauma evidenced by widening of the periodontal ligament space

    E. Radiographic appearance of health or gingivitis (American Academy of Periodontology Case Type I)

      1. Interproximal alveolar bone appears within 1.5 to 2 mm below the cemento-enamel junction.

      2. Lamina dura visible and radiopaque.

      3. Crestal bone pointed in the anterior region; horizontal and intersects the tooth at 90-degree angle in the posterior region.

    F. Radiographic appearance of slight chronic periodontitis (American Academy of Periodontology Case Type II)

      1. Loss of density in the alveolar crest area.

      2. Interproximal bone in the anterior region appears slightly less pointed; indistinct fuzziness in the posterior region.

      3. Triangulation may be present.

    G. Radiographic appearance of moderate chronic or aggressive periodontitis (American Academy of Periodontology Case Type III)

      1. Alveolar bone loss appears to be 30–50 percent when compared with the tooth root length.

      2. Crestal bone loss may be horizontally or vertically patterned.

      3. Radiolucencies between the roots of multirooted teeth may indicate furcation involvement.

    H. Radiographic appearance of advanced chronic or aggressive periodontitis (American Academy of Periodontology Case Type IV)

      1. Easily recognized radiographically.

      2. Alveolar bone loss appears to be greater than 50 percent when compared with the tooth root length.

      3. Furcation involvement is evident.

      4. Tooth movement may be evident radiographically as shifted or displaced teeth.

  V. Radiographic appearance of caries

    A. Advantages of the use of radiographs in the detection of caries.

      1. Images proximal surface caries that cannot be detected clinically.

      2. Images the extent of carious lesions.

B. Limitations of the use of radiographs in the detection of caries

      1. Caries are usually more advanced than the radiograph indicates.

      2. Occlusal, buccal, and lingual caries are not imaged until moderately advanced.

      3. Other conditions, such as abrasion, attrition, and radiolucent composite restorative materials may mimic caries.

      4. Optical illusions, such as cervical burnout and mach banding, interfere with caries detection.

C. Radiographic techniques

      1. Paralleling technique

        a. Parallel central ray of the x-ray beam images the proximal surface contact area more accurately than bisecting technique.

        b. Bitewing radiographs easily provide an accurate representation of the proximal surface contact area.

        c. Periapical radiographs require precise vertical angulation to achieve the accurate representation of the interproximal contact area achieved with bitewing radiographs.

      2. kVp

        a. Lower kVp setting produces a short scale (high contrast) image.

        b. High contrast will image subtle radiolucent changes in the radiopaque enamel.

D. Proximal surface caries

      1. Appear at or just apical to the proximal surface contact area

      2. When bone loss is present, may appear on the root surface

      3. Proximal surface caries grading system (suggested by Haugejorden and Slack, 1977)

        a. C-1 Incipient

          1) Appears as a radiolucent notch

          2) Penetrates less than halfway through the enamel

        b. C-2 Moderate

          1) Appears as a radiolucent triangle

          2) Penetrates more than halfway through the enamel but does not reach the dentin-enamel junction

        c. C-3 Advanced

          1) Appears as two radiolucent triangles

          2) Penetrates the dentin-enamel junction but does not reach more than halfway to the pulp

        d. C-4 Severe

          1) Appears as two radiolucent triangles or a large, diffuse radiolucency

          2) Penetrates the dentin-enamel junction and reaches more than halfway to the pulp

E. Buccal/lingual caries

      1. Appear as a round radiolucency in the center of the tooth crown

      2. Cannot differentiate between buccal and lingual location of carious lesion on a two-dimensional radiograph

F. Occlusal caries
   1. Appear as a radiolucency just apical to the occlusal enamel
   2. Usually not visible radiographically until moderately advanced
G. Root caries
   1. Appear as a notched or triangular-shaped radiolucency on the proximal surface at or below the cementoenamel junction.
   2. Bone loss is usually evident in the area, indicating an exposed root surface.
H. Recurrent decay
   1. Appears as a radiolucency adjacent to a restoration margin.
   2. Indirect pulp capping may mimic recurrent decay.
      a. Indirect pulp capping appears as a radiolucent shadow adjacent to a restoration.
      b. Indicates where a sedative base and permanent restoration were placed over decay that was not excavated to avoid exposing the pulp.
VI. Radiographic appearance of common oral pathologic conditions
   A. Advantages of the use of radiographs in the detection of common oral pathologic conditions
      1. Asymptomatic abnormalities detected
      2. Locates lesions that cannot be detected clinically
   B. Limitations of the use of radiographs in the detection of common oral pathologic conditions
      1. Radiographic findings should be utilized in conjunction with the clinical examination.
      2. Two-dimensional radiographs of three-dimensional structures may miss or mimic a pathologic condition.
   C. Pulpal changes
      1. Resorption
         a. Internal resorption
            1) Appears as a radiolucent widening of the pulp chamber.
            2) Differentiate from external resorption by the widening of the pulp chamber.
         b. External resorption
            1) Appears as shortened or blunted root structure when resorption begins at the apex
            2) May also appear as a round or diffuse radiolucency on the tooth root
            3) Differentiate from internal resorption by the unaffected root canal
      2. Pulp stone
         a. Appears as a radiopaque sphere in the pulp chamber
         b. Differentiate from enamel pearl by its location inside of the pulp chamber
      3. Pulpal sclerosis
         a. Appears as a narrowing or disappearance of the pulp chamber
         b. Appearance of secondary dentin
   D. Periapical lesions
      1. Radiolucent
         a. Abscess, cyst, granuloma

        1) Initially appear as a widening of the periodontal ligament space

        2) Develops into a circular radiolucency at the apex of the tooth

        3) Cannot be distinguished from each other with a radiograph alone

   b. Mental foramen (normal anatomy)

        1) May mimic an abscess or cyst especially when imaged at the root tip of the mandibular second or first premolar

        2) Differentiate from apical pathology by the location of the lamina dura and the periodontal ligament space.

           a) The lamina dura and the periodontal ligament space appear in the normal location, closely outlining the tooth root, when the observed radiolucency is the mental foramen.

           b) The lamina dura and the periodontal ligament space appear to extend away from the normal location, and do not closely outline the tooth root, but rather seem to outline the observed radiolucency when the most likely interpretation is apical pathology.

  2. Radiopaque

   a. Condensing osteitis

        1) Appears as a diffuse or circular radiopacity near the apices of a non-vital tooth.

        2) Differentiate from sclerotic bone by the history of prolonged inflammation associated with the tooth present.

        3) Differentiate from hypercementosis by the presence of the periodontal ligament space; condensing osteitis does not appear to be attached to the tooth.

   b. Sclerotic bone

        1) Appears as a diffuse or circular radiopacity not associated with prolonged inflammation of a tooth.

        2) Differentiate from condensing osteitis by the absence of chronic inflammation of the tooth present.

        3) Differentiate from hypercementosis by the presence of the periodontal ligament space; sclerotic bone does not appear to be attached to the tooth.

   c. Hypercementosis

        1) Appears as an overgrowth of cementum.

        2) Roots appear enlarged and bulbous.

        3) Differentiate between hypercementosis and condensing osteitis by the presence of the lamina dura and periodontal ligament space, which outline and surround the hypercementosis and separate the tooth root from the alveolar bone.

E. Other cysts

  1. Residual cyst

   a. Appears as a round, ovoid radiolucency

   b. Differentiates from other cysts by the location in an extraction site

2. Dentigerous cyst
   a. Appears as a round, ovoid radiolucency surrounding the crown only of an unerupted tooth
   b. Differentiate from the normal developing tooth and dental sac by the extent and size of the radiolucency
F. Periapical cemental dysplasia
   1. Early lesion appears radiolucent.
   2. Middle stage lesion appears as a mixed radiolucent and radiopaque mass.
   3. Mature lesion appears radiopaque with slight radiolucent "halo" effect.
   4. Usually located in the mandibular anterior region.
G. Odontoma
   1. Appears as a group of radiopaque toothlike lesions representing various formations of hard dental tissue (enamel, cementum, dentin)
   2. Usually associated with an unerupted tooth
H. Other conditions that may be observed on a radiograph
   1. Trauma
      a. Fracture appears as a radiolucent break in the root or crown of the tooth.
      b. Erosion appears as an increased radiolucency of the tooth crowns.
      c. Attrition appears as an increased radiolucency of the occlusal/incisal surface.
      d. Abrasion, when located near the cervical area, appears as a notched or triangular radiolucency that may mimic caries.
   2. Foreign materials
      a. Materials accidentally lodged in the soft or hard tissue, such as amalgam or orthodontic wires
      b. The presence of facial jewelry, such as tongue and lip piercing
      c. Metal objects appear radiopaque

BIBLIOGRAPHY

Frommer, HH, Stabulas-Savage, JJ. *Radiology for the Dental Professional,* 8th ed. St. Louis, MO: Elsevier; 2005: 436–446.

Haring, JI, Howerton, LJ. *Dental Radiography. Principles and Techniques,* 3rd ed. St. Louis, MO: Elsevier; 2006: 468–478.

Perry, DA, Beemsterboer P, Taggart, EJ. *Periodontology for the Dental Hygienist,* 2nd ed. St. Louis, MO: Elsevier; 2001: 176–181.

Reddy, M. Radiographic methods for the detection of progressive alveolar bone loss. *Journal of Periodontology.* 1992; 63:1078–1084.

Reed, B, Polson, A. Relationships between bitewing and periapical radiographs in assessing crestal alveolar bone levels. *Journal of Periodontology.* 1984; 55:22–27.

Thomson, EM, Tolle, L. A practical guide for using radiographs in the assessment of periodontal diseases. Part I: technique. *Practical Hygiene.* 1994; 3:11–16.

1. All of the following are useful aids for interpretation of dental radiographs *except* one. Which one is this *exception?*
   - A. Viewbox
   - B. Magnifying glass
   - C. Bright room lighting
   - D. Film mount

2. Your patient's maxillary anterior periapical radiograph reveals shorter than normal root lengths on the maxillary lateral incisor. Which of the following is the most likely interpretation?
   - A. External resorption
   - B. Microdontia
   - C. Pulpal sclerosis
   - D. Root fracture

3. A 63-year-old patient has no symptoms. A mandibular periapical radiograph reveals ovoid radiopacities located in the pulp chambers of the mandibular molars. Which of the following is the most likely interpretation?
   - A. Cysts
   - B. Hyperdontia
   - C. Pulp stones
   - D. Supernumerary teeth

4. Which of the following dental materials would appear *radiolucent* radiographically?
   - A. Acrylic
   - B. Amalgam
   - C. Implant
   - D. Metallic crown

5. Which of the following is a *limitation* of radiographs in evaluating periodontal disease?
   - A. Estimating bone loss
   - B. Locating irritants
   - C. Determining prognosis
   - D. Differentiating between active and inactive disease status

6. An early periodontal health change is seen radiographically as
   - A. An enlargement of the gingiva
   - B. Furcation involvement
   - C. Loss of density of alveolar crest
   - D. Vertical bone loss

7. All of the following may resemble caries radiographically *except* one. Which one is this *exception?*
   - A. Abrasion
   - B. Attrition
   - C. Cervical burnout
   - D. Metallic restoration

8. Interproximal carious lesions frequently appear radiographically on which area of the tooth?
   A. At or just apical to the occlusal/incisal edge
   B. At or just apical to the gingival margin
   C. At or just apical to the proximal contact area
   D. At or just apical to the CEJ

9. A periapical abscess and a periapical cyst can be differentiated on a radiograph by
   A. Whether or not lesion margins are diffuse or well demarcated.
   B. The presence or absence of associated tooth root resorption.
   C. The size and shape of the radiolucency.
   D. Abscess and cysts cannot be differentiated from the radiograph alone.

10. A radiolucent oval seen near the apex of the mandibular second premolars that may mimic periapical pathology is
    A. Cervical burnout
    B. Lingual foramen
    C. Mandibular foramen
    D. Mental foramen

laboratory exercise 13

Supplemental Radiographic Techniques

INTRODUCTION

A dental radiographer must possess the knowledge and skills to perform basic oral radiographic techniques. What sets the exceptional dental radiographer apart is the ability to adapt techniques to perform advanced radiographic services for the patient. Theory provides the knowledge base that guides radiographic practice, but acceptable deviations from the basic techniques, when implemented correctly, can obtain radiographs in situations that might have made radiographs unobtainable. In addition to acquiring quality radiographs under less than ideal conditions, the dental radiographer trained in advanced techniques can interpret the maximum amount of information from radiographs.

The purpose of this exercise is to introduce the student to three specialized dental radiographic skills. Practicing these skills and evaluating the resulting images will complete the competent dental radiographer's skill set.

OBJECTIVES

Following completion of this lab activity, you will be able to:

1. Demonstrate proficiency in placing, exposing, and processing topographical and cross-sectional occlusal radiographs.

2. Demonstrate proficiency in placing, exposing, and processing disto-oblique periapical radiographs.

3. Demonstrate proficiency in applying two methods of localization: right-angle and tube-shift.

4. Identify the buccal/lingual positions of objects radiographically utilizing a localization method.

325

MATERIALS

Teaching manikin or skull

Lead (or lead-equivalent) apron with thyroid collar

Size #2 radiographic films

Size #4 radiographic films

Periapical film-holding device

Metal object or sample extracted tooth

Lead letters "M," "D," "O," and "A" or similar metal objects for labeling

Red sticky wax or similar adhesive material

View box

PREPARATION

1. Study the chapter outline to prepare for this laboratory exercise. An understanding of the material presented in the outline is required to complete this activity.

2. Utilize Tables 13.1 and 13.2 to assist you with completing the exercises. Instructor demonstration may enhance knowledge of the laboratory exercise.

3. Prepare radiology operatory. Set up teaching manikin or skull. Ensure that correct "patient" positioning is achieved for the type of projection you are exposing. To image the maxilla, ensure that the maxillary occlusal plane is parallel to the floor; to image the mandible, ensure that the mandibular occlusal plane is parallel to the floor and the midsagittal plane must be perpendicular to the floor for both maxillary and mandibular exposures. Tip the patient's head back so that the occlusal plane is perpendicular to the floor for the mandibular cross-sectional occlusal radiographs

4. Place lead apron (or lead-equivalent barrier) and thyroid collar over the "patient."

LABORATORY EXERCISE ACTIVITIES

Part 1: Occlusal Radiographs

1. Obtain five size #4 radiographic film packets.

2. Check posted exposure settings for the dental x-ray unit, and set for occlusal radiographs. (If no setting for occlusal radiographs are posted, use the settings for periapical radiographs in that region.)

3. Using Table 13.1, place and expose the following occlusal radiographs:
   a. Maxillary anterior topographical occlusal radiograph
   b. Maxillary posterior topographical occlusal radiograph (Choose either the right or the left side.)
   c. Mandibular anterior topographical occlusal radiograph

TABLE 13.1   Occlusal Radiographs

Occlusal Radiograph	Film Packet Placement	Vertical Angulation	Horizontal Angulation	Centering
Maxillary topographical (anterior)	Long dimension across the mouth (buccal-to-buccal). White unprinted side toward the maxillary teeth.	Direct the central rays perpendicular to the imaginary bisector between the long axes of the teeth and the film in the vertical dimension; +65 degrees	Direct the central rays of the x-ray beam perpendicular to patient's midsagittal plane; through the maxillary central incisors interproximal space.	Direct the central rays of the x-ray beam through a point near the bridge of the nose toward the center of the film.
Maxillary topographical (posterior)	Long dimension along the midline (front-to-back). White unprinted side toward the maxillary teeth.	Direct the central rays perpendicular to the imaginary bisector between the long axes of the teeth and the film in the vertical dimension; +45 degrees	Direct the central rays of the x-ray beam perpendicular to patient's midsagittal plane; through the maxillary first and second molar interproximal space.	Direct the central rays of the x-ray beam through a point on on the cheek bone below the outer cantus (corner) of the eye toward the center of the film.
Mandibular topographical (anterior)	Long dimension across the mouth (buccal-to-buccal). White unprinted side toward the mandibular teeth.	Direct the central rays perpendicular to the imaginary bisector between the long axes of the teeth and the film in the vertical dimension; −55 degrees	Direct the central rays of the x-ray beam perpendicular to patient's midsagittal plane; through the mandibular central incisors interproximal space.	Direct the central rays of the x-ray beam through a point in the middle of the chin toward the center of the film.
Mandibular topographical (posterior)	Long dimension along the midline (front-to-back). White unprinted side toward the mandibular teeth.	Direct the central rays perpendicular to the imaginary bisector between the long axes of the teeth and the film in the vertical dimension; −45 degrees	Direct the central rays of the x-ray beam perpendicular to patient's midsagittal plane through the mandibular first and second molar interproximal space.	Direct the central rays of the x-ray beam through a point on the inferior border of the mandible directly below the second mandibular premolar toward the center of the film.
Mandibular cross-sectional	Long dimension across the mouth (buccal-to-buccal). White unprinted side toward the mandibular teeth.	Direct the central rays perpendicular to the film; 0 degrees	Direct the central rays of the x-ray beam perpendicular to patient's midsagittal plane through the middle of the sublingual region.	Direct the central rays of the x-ray beam through a point 2 in. (5 cm) back from the tip of the chin toward the center of the film.

Modified from Johnson, ON, Thomson, EM. *Essentials of Dental Radiography for Dental Assistants and Hygienists,* 8th ed., Upper Saddle River, NJ: Prentice Hall: 2007: 212.

TABLE 13.2 Disto-Oblique Periapical Radiographs

Maxillary Disto-Oblique Periapical Radiograph	Mandibular Disto-Oblique Periapical Radiograph
Position the film packet as far posteriorly as possible.	Position the film packet as far posteriorly as possible.
Align the PID into the correct vertical and horizontal angles for a standard periapical radiograph. Center the film packet in the middle of the x-ray beam.	Align the PID into the correct vertical and horizontal angles for a standard periapical radiograph. Center the film packet in the middle of the x-ray beam.
Alter the horizontal angulation by shifting the PID so that the x-ray beam will intersect the film 10 degrees from the distal.	Alter the horizontal angulation by shifting the PID so that the x-ray beam will intersect the film 10 degrees from the distal.
Increase the horizontal angulation 10 degrees over standard.	Do not change the horizontal angulation from standard.
Increase the exposure time by one impulse setting over standard.	Do not change the exposure time from standard .

    d. Mandibular posterior topographical occlusal radiograph (Choose either the right or the left side.)

    e. Mandibular cross-sectional occlusal radiograph (Reposition the "patient's" head by tipping the chin up.)

  4. Process the five films.

Part 2: Disto-Oblique Periapical Radiographs

1. Using red sticky wax or other adhesive, attach an extracted molar or metal object to the teaching manikin or skull in the area of the maxillary tuberosity (Figure 13.1 ■) and in the region of the mandibular retro-molar pad (Figure 13.2 ■). (Use the patient's right side for this exercise.) This object will simulate a posteriorly located impaction or foreign object.

2. Obtain four size #2 radiographic film packets.

3. Check the posted exposure settings for the dental x-ray unit, and set for a maxillary molar periapical radiograph.

4. Using a film holder and the paralleling technique, place the first film packet in the *standard* film packet position for exposing the maxillary right molar periapical. (Note that this standard position will *not* image the posteriorly located impacted molar or metal object. This would be especially true if this patient had a hypersensitive gag reflex, which would prevent posterior placement of the film packet.)

5. Expose the standard maxillary molar periapical and set aside.

6. Next, check the posted exposure settings for the dental x-ray unit, and set for a mandibular molar periapical radiograph.

7. Using the paralleling technique, place the second film packet in the *standard* film packet position for exposing the mandibular right molar

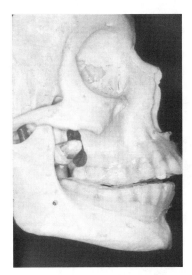

Figure 13.1 A posteriorly located "impacted" maxillary molar is attached to the teaching manikin with sticky wax.

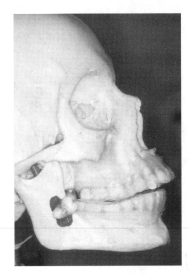

Figure 13.2 A posteriorly located "impacted" mandibular molar is attached to the teaching manikin with sticky wax.

periapical. (This standard position will *not* image the posteriorly located impacted molar or metal object.)

8. Then use Table 13.2 to place and expose the following:
   a. Maxillary disto-oblique periapical radiograph
   b. Mandibular disto-oblique periapical radiograph

9. Place the film packets for the disto-oblique periapical exposures in the *exact same* position as the *standard* film packets were placed when you exposed the maxillary and mandibular right molar periapicals. (Again, this standard position will *not* image the posteriorly located "impacted" molar or metal object.)

10. Process the four films.

Part 3: Right-Angle Method of Localization

1. Using red sticky wax or other adhesive, attach an extracted molar or metal object to the teaching manikin or skull on the buccal side of the

Supplemental Radiographic Techniques **329**

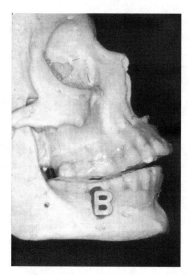

Figure 13.3 A metal object is attached to the teaching manikin with sticky wax to simulate the presence of a foreign body.

right mandibular first molar region (Figure 13.3 ■) and the lingual side of the left mandibular first molar region. Center the objects in the middle of the furcation area of the first molars. These objects will simulate an impaction or foreign object.

2. Obtain two size #2 and one size #4 radiographic film packets.

3. Check the posted exposure settings for the dental x-ray unit, and set for mandibular posterior periapical radiographs.

4. Using a film holder and the two size #2 film packets, place and expose the mandibular right and the mandibular left molar periapical radiographs utilizing the paralleling technique. Set aside.

5. Reposition the patient's head for exposing a mandibular cross-sectional occlusal radiograph.

6. Check posted exposure settings for the dental x-ray unit, and set for the mandibular cross-sectional occlusal radiograph.

7. Using Table 13.1 and the size #4 film packet, place and expose the mandibular cross-sectional occlusal radiograph.

8. Process the three films.

Part 4: Tube-Shift Method of Localization

1. Attach an extracted molar or metal object to the buccal side of the mandibular right first molar region and to the lingual side of the mandibular left first molar region. Use the same positions for the objects that you used in Part 3. (Figure 13.3)

2. Obtain ten size #2 radiographic film packets.

3. Check the posted exposure settings for the dental x-ray unit, and set for mandibular posterior periapical radiographs.

4. Obtain a periapical film holder. Use a device such as a Stabe film holder without an extension arm and aiming device, since these may get in the way when altering the angulation of the PID.

5. Using two of the size #2 film packets, place and expose standard mandibular right and mandibular left molar periapical radiographs utilizing the paralleling technique. Set aside.

6. Next, use four more size #2 film packets to expose the mandibular right molar. The film packet position should be the same as the standard placement, only, now, you will be shifting the PID from standard alignment. Using sticky wax, label each of the four films you will be using with a lead letter so that you will be able to identify which image was taken with which shift in the PID alignment. Place the lead letter near the edge of the film packet to position it out of the way (Figure 13.4 ■).

7. Shift the PID horizontally and vertically, into the following four positions for each of the four exposures on the right side. Obtain an additional four films and repeat this step with each of the four exposures on the left side. Shift the PID:

   a. Horizontally, so that the x-ray beam will strike the film 10 degrees from the mesial. (Label film with the lead letter "M.") (Figure 13.5 ■)

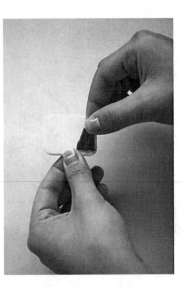

Figure 13.4 Labeling the film packet by attaching a lead letter with sticky wax.

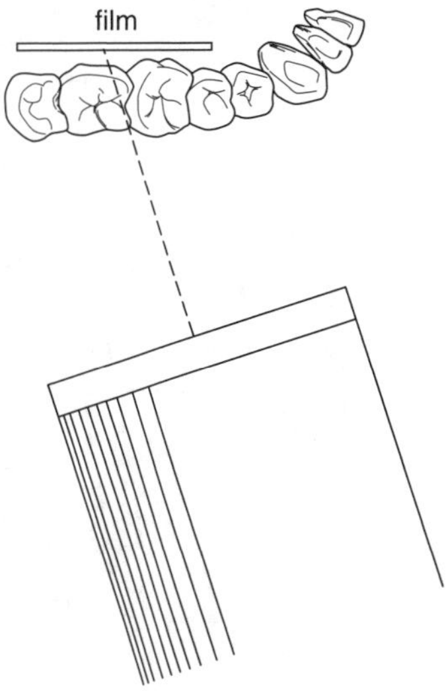

film

Figure 13.5 Tube-shift method of localization exercise. Alter the horizontal angulation approximately 10 degrees from the mesial.

b. Horizontally, so that the x-ray beam will strike the film 10 degrees from the distal. (Label film with the lead letter "D.") (Figure 13.6 ■)

c. Vertically, so that the x-ray beam will strike the film 10 degrees from the occlusal plane. (Label film with the lead letter "O.") (Figure 13.7 ■)

d. Vertically, so that the x-ray beam will strike the film 10 degrees from the apical region. (Label film with the lead letter "A.") (Figure 13.8 ■)

8. Process the films exposed on the right side first, or separately from the films exposed on the left side to avoid mixing them up.

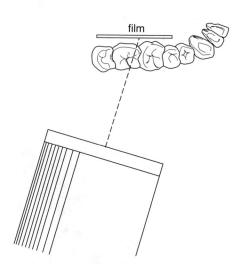

Figure 13.6 Tube-shift method of localization exercise. Alter the horizontal angulation approximately 10 degrees from the distal.

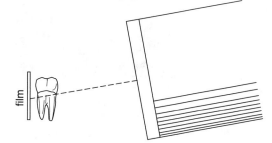

Figure 13.7 Tube-shift method of localization exercise. Alter the vertical angulation approximately 10 degrees from the occlusal.

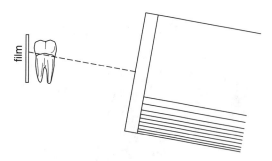

Figure 13.8 Tube-shift method of localization exercise. Alter the vertical angulation approximately 10 degrees from the apical.

COMPETENCY AND EVALUATION

1. Mount the processed films on the simulated film mounts that follow. Secure with a piece of tape placed along the top edge of the film only, so that the films may be raised slightly, to allow light underneath for ease of viewing.

   NOTE: Use the labial mounting method. (See Laboratory Exercise 8, Film Mounting and Radiographic Landmarks, for details.) The raised portion of the embossed dot is toward you (convex) when placing the film onto the page.

2. Place the simulated mount pages on a viewbox and evaluate. Obtain instructor feedback.

3. Examine the resultant radiographic images in each of the four parts of this exercise. Based on your results, summarize the following in your own words:

   a. Part 1 Occlusal Radiographs
      Describe the difference in appearance between the image obtained utilizing the topographical technique and the cross-sectional technique. What conditions might the patient present with that would prompt the dentist to prescribe a topographical occlusal radiograph? A cross-sectional occlusal radiograph? Based on the four steps: packet placement, vertical and horizontal angulation, and centering the PID, what is the quality of the images? Are the correct teeth imaged? Is there elongation or foreshortening error? Is the area of interest overlapped? Is there cone-cut error? Does the cone-cut affect an important part of the image? Why would cone-cut error be acceptable in the anterior region of the image? What steps would you take to improve your skills in taking occlusal radiographs?

   b. Part 2 Disto-Oblique Periapical Radiographs
      Compare the standard and disto-oblique periapical radiographs side-by-side. Is the disto-oblique image a reasonable representation of the anatomical structures? Is image distortion minimal? Describe the difference between the two images. Did the disto-oblique image structures that were located further posteriorly than the film placement could access? What is the advantage to this? What conditions might the patient present with that would prompt the dentist to prescribe a disto-oblique periapical radiograph?

   c. Part 3 Right-Angle Method of Localization
      Describe the role the cross-sectional occlusal radiograph plays in locating buccal-lingual objects radiographically. Why would it be difficult to utilize occlusal radiographs to locate objects on the maxilla?

   d. If you did not know where these objects were attached, how would you be able to tell the buccal or lingual location by examining these films? When examining the radiographs of the right side, what can you summarize about the direction the object appeared to "move"? When examining the radiographs of the left side, what can you summarize about the direction the object appeared to "move"? Explain how you would utilize your knowledge of the tube-shift method of locating an object imaged in two places on a full mouth or bitewing series?

4. Complete the study questions.

Part 1: Occlusal Radiographs

Maxillary Anterior Topographical

Maxillary Posterior Topographical

Mandibular Anterior Topographical

Mandibular Posterior Topographical

Mandibular Cross-Sectional

Part 2: Disto-Oblique Periapical Radiographs

Maxillary Standard Periapical   Maxillary Disto-Oblique Periapical

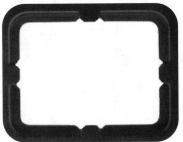

Mandibular Standard Periapical   Mandibular Disto-Oblique Periapical

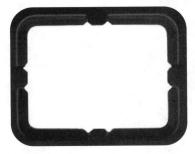

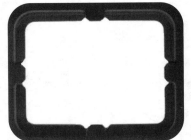

Part 3: Right Angle Localization Method

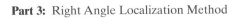

Standard Periapical
of Buccal Object

Standard Periapical
of Lingual Object

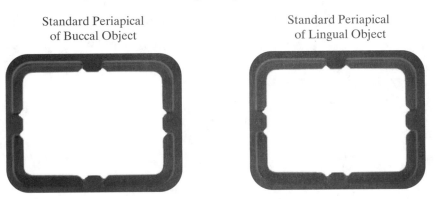

Occlusal Cross Sectional (right angle projection)

Part 4: Tube Shift Method of Localization—Buccal Location

Occlusal PID shift

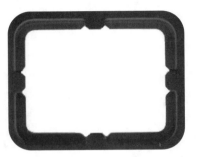

Distal PID shift   Standard periapical   Mesial PID shift

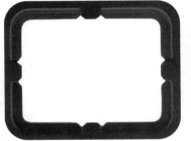 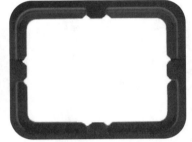 

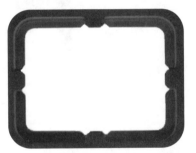

Apical PID shift

Part 4: Tube Shift Method of Localization—Lingual Location

Occlusal PID shift

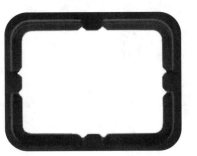

Distal PID shift

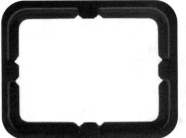

Standard periapical

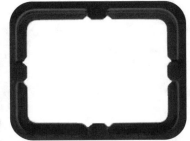

Mesial PID shift

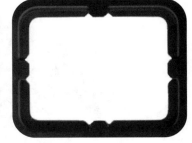

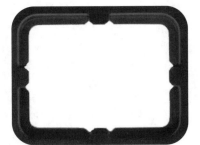

Apical PID shift

I. Occlusal radiographs
   A. Purpose
      1. Image a larger area than periapical radiographs
      2. Can be used as an acceptable substitute when the patient cannot tolerate intraoral placement of periapical radiographs (Figure 13.9 ■)
         a. Children
         b. Patients with a low, sensitive palatal vault
         c. Patients with an exaggerated gag reflex
         d. Patients who are unable to open due to fractures or temporomandibular disorder (TMD)
      3. Can be used as an aid in locating the buccal or lingual position of foreign objects, impactions, or supernumerary teeth, cysts, or other conditions
   B. Technique
      1. Utilizes size #4 radiographic film.
      2. Size #2 film may be used with the occlusal technique for the child patient.
      3. Technique is based on bisecting technique, where the central ray of the x-ray beam is directed perpendicular to the imaginary bisector between the long axes of the teeth and the film packet plane.
      4. The white, unprinted side of the film packet is placed toward the arch being imaged.
      5. The embossed dot is placed away from the area of interest (toward the anterior). (Figure 13.10 ■)
      6. The film packet should extend at least one-fourth inch beyond the anterior teeth of the arch image imaged. (Figure 13.10)
      7. Unit settings should be based on the manufacturer's recommendations.
   C. Maxillary anterior topographical occlusal radiograph
      1. Seat the patient upright with occlusal plane parallel to the floor and the mid-saggital plane perpendicular to the floor.
      2. Place the film packet with the long dimension horizontal, across the patient's right and left sides.
      3. Direct the horizontal angulation perpendicular to the film through the maxillary central incisors.

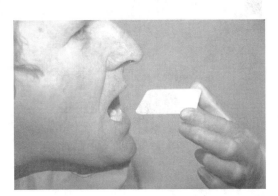

Figure 13.9 The occlusal film packet placement is easily tolerated by the patient with a low, sensitive palatal vault.

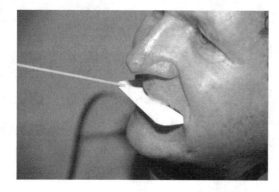

Figure 13.10 The embossed dot is placed anteriorly and the film packet is extending at least one-fourth inch beyond the maxillary anterior teeth, indicating correct maxillary topographical occlusal film packet placement.

4. Align the vertical angulation perpendicular to the imaginary bisector of the long axes plane of the teeth and the film packet plane or at approximately +65 degrees through a point at the bridge of the nose. (Figure 13.11 ■)
5. Center the film in the x-ray beam to avoid cone-cutting the image.

D. Maxillary posterior topographical occlusal radiograph
1. Seat the patient upright with occlusal plane parallel to the floor and the midsagittal plane perpendicular to the floor.
2. Place the film packet with the long dimension vertical, along the patient's midline over the quadrant being imaged.
3. Direct the horizontal angulation perpendicular to the film through the maxillary first molar and the maxillary second premolar interproximal space.
4. Align the vertical angulation perpendicular to the imaginary bisector of the long axes plane of the teeth and the film packet plane or at approximately +45 degrees through the outer canthus (corner) of the eye. (Figure 13.12 ■)
5. Center the film in the x-ray beam to avoid cone-cutting the image.

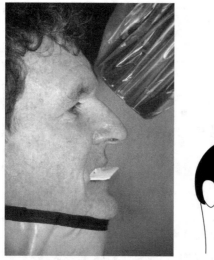

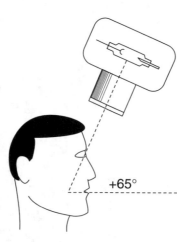

+65°

Figure 13.11 Vertical angulation required for the maxillary anterior topographical occlusal radiograph.

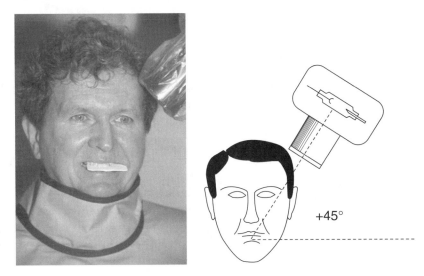

Figure 13.12 Vertical angulation required for the maxillary posterior topographical occlusal radiograph.

+45°

E. Mandibular anterior topographical occlusal radiograph
   1. Seat the patient upright with occlusal plane parallel to the floor and the midsagittal plane perpendicular to the floor.
   2. Place the film packet with the long dimension horizontal, across the patient's right and left sides.
   3. Direct the horizontal angulation perpendicular to the film through the mandibular central incisors.
   4. Align the vertical angulation perpendicular to the imaginary bisector of the long axes plane of the teeth and the film packet plane or at approximately −55 degrees through the inferior border of the mandible, at the midpoint of the chin. (Figure 13.13 ■)
   5. Center the film in the x-ray beam to avoid cone-cutting the image.

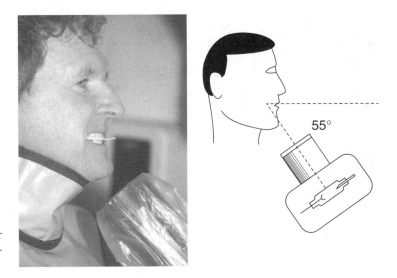

55°

Figure 13.13 Vertical angulation required for the mandibular anterior topographical occlusal radiograph.

F. Mandibular posterior topographical occlusal radiograph
1. Seat the patient upright with occlusal plane parallel to the floor and the mid-sagittal plane perpendicular to the floor.
2. Place the film packet with the long dimension vertical, along the patient's midline over the quadrant being imaged.
3. Direct the horizontal angulation perpendicular to the film through the mandibular first molar and the mandibular second premolar interproximal space.
4. Align the vertical angulation perpendicular to the imaginary bisector of the long axes plane of the teeth and the film packet plane or at approximately −45 degrees through the inferior border of the mandible apical to the mandibular second premolar. (Figure 13.14 ■)
5. Center the film in the x-ray beam to avoid cone-cutting the image.

G. Mandibular cross-sectional occlusal radiograph
1. Seat the patient upright with the chin up and the head tilted back as far as possible to align the occlusal plane perpendicular to the floor.
2. Place the film packet with the long dimension horizontal, across the patient's right and left sides.
3. Direct the horizontal angulation perpendicular to the film through the mandibular sublingual area.
4. Align the vertical angulation perpendicular to the film. (Figure 13.15 ■) When the patient is seated correctly the vertical angulation on the tube head will read 0 degrees.
5. Center the film in the x-ray beam to avoid cone-cutting the image.

H. Criteria for acceptance
1. Area of interest is accurately imaged on the film.
2. No overlapping of the proximal surfaces.
3. Image is free of distortion (elongation or foreshortening).

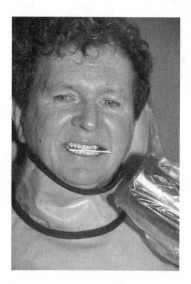

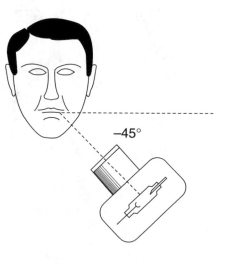

−45°

Figure 13.14 Vertical angulation required for the mandibular posterior topographical occlusal radiograph.

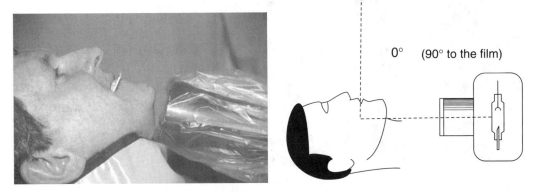

0° (90° to the film)

Figure 13.15 Vertical angulation required for the mandibular cross-sectional occlusal radiograph.

4. Cone-cutting is absent or minimal. (If cone-cutting occurs, it should be confined to the anterior region of the film where no image is affected.)
5. Embossed dot should be away from the image area, positioned toward the anterior region.

II. Disto-oblique periapical radiographs
  A. Purpose
    1. Allows imagery in the posterior region with minimal discomfort for the patient
    2. May eliminate the need for an extraoral dental radiograph
  B. Uses
    1. Images distally located supernumerary teeth or foreign objects located in the maxillary tuberosity area or the region of the mandibular retro-molar pad (Figure 13.16 ■)
    2. Allows imagery in the posterior region of the patient with a hypersensitive gag reflex
  C. Limitations
    1. Increased image distortion results from an alteration in the vertical angulation.
    2. Increased overlapping of the proximal surfaces results from an alteration in the horizontal angulation.
    3. Image distortion and overlapping are acceptable to achieve the goal of imaging a posteriorly located object (Figure 13.16).
  D. Technique
    1. Utilizes the same size film as used for a standard periapical radiograph.
    2. The horizontal angulation is altered to project the image of the posteriorly located object anteriorly onto the film.

Figure 13.16 A comparison of a standard maxillary molar periapical radiograph (left) and a maxillary disto-oblique periapical radiograph (right). Note the increase in posterior imagery achieved with the disto-oblique periapical radiograph. The increased image distortion and overlap in the disto-oblique periapical radiograph is considered acceptable when utilizing this technique.

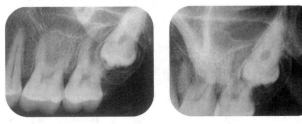

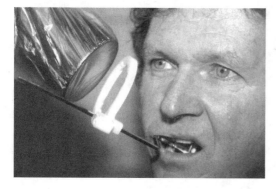

Figure 13.17 Beam alignment for a maxillary disto-oblique periapical radiograph demonstrating how the PID and the external aiming device of the film holder are no longer aligned. Note that altering the horizontal angulation approximately 10 degrees can be estimated by directing the PID approximately 1 to 2 inches from standard.

    3. The vertical angulation is altered for the maxillary disto-oblique periapical radiograph to project the apically located object down onto the film.

    4. When using a film holder with an external aiming device such as the Rinn XCP instrument, the P.I.D. and the ring will no longer align with each other. (Figure 13.17 ■)

E. Maxillary disto-oblique periapical radiograph

    1. The patient is seated upright with occlusal plane parallel to the floor and the mid-saggital plane perpendicular to the floor.

    2. Utilizing the paralleling technique, the film packet is placed as far posteriorly as possible.

    3. The horizontal and vertical angulations are directed as for a standard maxillary posterior periapical radiograph. (See Laboratory Exercise 3, Periapical Radiographs—Paralleling Technique.)

    4. From this standard alignment, the PID is shifted horizontally to direct the x-ray beam to intersect the film obliquely 10 degrees from the distal. (Figure 13.17)

    5. From the standard vertical alignment, the PID is shifted vertically to direct the x-ray beam to intersect the film obliquely at an angulation that is increased by 5 degrees.

    6. The standard exposure time used for a maxillary posterior periapical radiograph is increased by one impulse setting over that standard setting to allow for the oblique penetration of the x-ray beam through the zygoma in this altered position.

F. Mandibular disto-oblique periapical radiograph

    1. The patient is seated upright with the occlusal plane parallel to the floor and the mid-saggital plane perpendicular to the floor.

    2. Utilizing the paralleling technique, the film packet is placed as far posteriorly as possible.

    3. The horizontal and vertical angulations are directed as for a standard mandibular posterior periapical radiograph. (See Laboratory Exercise 3, Periapical Radiographs—Paralleling Technique.)

    4. From this standard alignment, the PID is shifted horizontally to direct the x-ray beam to intersect the film obliquely 10 degrees from the distal.

    5. No change in the vertical angulation is required for the mandibular disto-oblique periapical radiograph.

    6. No change in the exposure time setting is required for the mandibular disto-oblique periapical radiograph.

III. Localization
   A. Purpose
      1. Adds a third dimension to two-dimensional radiographs
      2. Used to determine the buccal or lingual position of an object radiographically
   B. Uses
      1. Locates the relative position of impactions
      2. Identifies the location of supernumerary teeth
      3. Aids in locating amalgam scrap, broken dental instruments, metallic fragments from accidents
      4. Aids endodontic therapy in determining the number and location of root canals
   C. Technique
      1. Utilizes the same size film as used for a standard periapical radiograph.
      2. The radiographic image of the object is observed following an alteration in the horizontal or vertical angulation.
      3. Comparing horizontal or vertical beam direction changes with a resulting image shift determines the buccal or lingual position of the object.
   D. Definitive-evaluation method of localization
      1. Relies on the shadow cast principle that states that the closer an object is to the film, the sharper the image definition. (See Laboratory Exercise 9, Exposure Variables—Factors Affecting the Radiographic Image.)
      2. Requires the exposure of only one film.
      3. Because the film is positioned lingually in the patient's oral cavity, an object located lingually will appear more sharply defined than an object located buccally.
      4. Least reliable method of localization.
   E. Right-angle method of localization
      1. Utilizes a cross-sectional occlusal radiograph to determine the buccal-lingual position of an object.
      2. Once an object has been identified on a standard radiograph, an additional exposure using the cross-sectional occlusal technique is required.
      3. More effective on the mandible than the maxilla.
      4. Requires an additional exposure.
   F. Tube-shift method of localization
      1. Utilizes the buccal-object rule.
         a. When two objects are in a straight line with the radiographer, one of the objects will be obscured from view.
         b. If the radiographer moves to the right, the more *distant* object will "move" into view by appearing to shift to the right.
         c. If the radiographer moves to the right, the *nearer* object will "move" to the left, revealing the more distant object.
      2. S.L.O.B. rule
         a. Objects that appear to move in the same direction as the PID shift are on the lingual—"Same on Lingual."
         b. Objects that appear to move in the opposite direction as the PID shift are on the buccal—"Opposite on Buccal."

3. Lingual objects
   a. When the PID shifts to direct the x-ray beam to intersect the film from the mesial, the object will appear to "move" toward the mesial.
   b. When the PID shifts to direct the x-ray beam to intersect the film from the distal, the object will appear to "move" toward the distal.
   c. When the PID shifts to direct the x-ray beam to intersect the film from the occlusal plane, the object will appear to "move" toward the occlusal.
   d. When the PID shifts to direct the x-ray beam to intersect the film from the apical region, the object will appear to "move" toward the apical.
4. Buccal objects
   a. When the PID shifts to direct the x-ray beam to intersect the film from the mesial, the object will appear to "move" toward the distal.
   b. When the PID shifts to direct the x-ray beam to intersect the film from the distal, the object will appear to "move" toward the mesial.
   c. When the PID shifts to direct the x-ray beam to intersect the film from the occlusal plane, the object will appear to "move" toward the apical.
   d. When the PID shifts to direct the x-ray beam to intersect the film from the apical region, the object will appear to "move" toward the occlusal.
5. May not require the exposure of an additional film, if the object has been imaged more than once, as in the case of a full mouth or bitewing series of radiographs

BIBLIOGRAPHY

Frommer, HH, Stabulas-Savage, JJ. *Radiology for the Dental Professional.*, 8th ed. St. Louis, MO: Elsevier; 2005: 251-258, 365-370.

Mauriello, SM, Overman, VP, Platin, E. *Radiographic Imaging for the Dental Team.* Philadelphia, PA: Lippincott Williams & Wilkins; 1995: 221-237.

O'Carroll, MK. *Advanced Radiographic Techniques Part I: Occlusal and Lateral Oblique Projections.* Study guide to videotape series. Chapel Hill, NC: Health Sciences Consortium; 1993.

1. Which of the following projections would *best* image an unexplained sublingual swelling?
   - A. Topographical occlusal radiograph
   - B. Cross-sectional occlusal radiograph
   - C. Disto-oblique periapical radiograph

2. Which of the following projections would *best* image an impacted maxillary third molar?
   - A. Topographical occlusal radiograph
   - B. Cross-sectional occlusal radiograph
   - C. Disto-oblique periapical radiograph

3. Which of the following projections would *best* evaluate delayed eruption of the maxillary lateral incisors in a child patient?
   - A. Topographical occlusal radiograph
   - B. Cross-sectional occlusal radiograph
   - C. Disto-oblique periapical radiograph

4. When placing a size #4 film for an occlusal radiograph, the embossed dot should be placed toward the
   - A. mesial
   - B. distal
   - C. posterior
   - D. anterior

5. For a maxillary disto-oblique periapical radiograph, the vertical angulation is _____ that used for the standard periapical radiograph.
   - A. increased by 5 degrees over
   - B. decreased by 5 degrees under
   - C. increased by 10 degrees over
   - D. decreased by 10 degrees under

6. For a mandibular disto-oblique periapical radiograph, the horizontal angulation is directed so that x-ray beam will strike the film obliquely _____.
   - A. 5 degrees from the distal
   - B. 5 degrees from the mesial
   - C. 10 degrees from the distal
   - D. 10 degrees from the mesial

7. For a mandibular disto-oblique periapical radiograph, the exposure setting should be _____.
   - A. increased by one impulse setting over the standard setting
   - B. decreased by one impulse setting over the standard setting
   - C. the same as the standard setting

8. Which of the following is the least reliable method of localization?
   - A. Definitive-evaluation method
   - B. Right-angle method
   - C. Tube-shift method

9. Referring to Part 4—Tube-Shift Method of Localization performed on the right side of the patient, when the PID shifted to direct the x-ray beam to intersect the film obliquely from the mesial, the object appeared to shift to the _____.
    A. mesial
    B. distal
    C. occlusal
    D. apical

10. Referring to Part 4—Tube-Shift Method of Localization performed on the left side of the patient, when the PID shifted to direct the x-ray beam to intersect the film obliquely from the mesial, the object appeared to shift to the _____.
    A. mesial
    B. distal
    C. occlusal
    D. apical

laboratory exercise 14

Panoramic Radiographic Technique

INTRODUCTION

There are situations when intraoral radiographs may not provide enough information about a patient's oral condition. Additionally, the patient may present with conditions that make intraoral film packet placement intolerable. The panoramic radiograph is the most commonly used extraoral dental radiographic technique. Although not a substitute for an intraoral radiographic examination, the panoramic radiograph plays a valuable role in assessing and diagnosing oral conditions. A panoramic radiograph may be exposed in less time, with minimal patient cooperation, and at a reduced dose of radiation when compared with a full mouth series of intraoral radiographs.

Although panoramic radiography is relatively simple to perform, the dental radiographer must possess certain skills to achieve quality diagnostic imaging. Most dental panoramic x-ray units offer manufacturer's recommendations to achieve quality imagery. However, there are key steps for exposing panoramic radiographs which are common to most all units. Knowledge of these key points not only will allow the dental radiographer to produce quality radiographic images on any machine, but also will aid the radiographer in applying corrective measures to less than ideal imagery.

The purpose of this laboratory exercise is to familiarize the student with the basic steps required for panoramic radiography and to provide the student with an opportunity to practice the procedure. Not all panoramic x-ray machines operate exactly the same; however, achieving a quality panoramic radiograph may be accomplished through an understanding of six key steps: (1) cassette and film preparation and care, (2) unit preparation, (3) patient preparation, (4) patient positioning, (5) exposure; and (6) processing. Practice of this laboratory exercise is on a student partner. Together, the student partners will simulate preparing a panoramic film and cassette for exposure and set up the panoramic x-ray unit. Patient preparation and positioning will be practiced on each other, establishing a real-life setting in which to become familiar with the operation of the panoramic equipment.

355

OBJECTIVES

Following completion of this lab activity, you will be able to:

1. Demonstrate proficiency in preparing the panoramic film and cassette for exposure.

2. Demonstrate correct patient positioning to achieve a quality panoramic radiograph.

3. Identify and apply corrective methods for common film care and handling, unit preparation, patient preparation and positioning, exposure, and processing errors which compromise the quality of a panoramic radiograph.

MATERIALS

Panoramic x-ray unit

Panoramic cassette with intensifying screens and practice film

Student partner

Lead (or lead-equivalent) apron with no thyroid collar attached

Hand washing station with antimicrobial soap or antiseptic hand rub

Disinfectant

Paper towels

Heavy duty utility gloves

PREPARATION

1. Study the chapter outline to prepare for this laboratory exercise. An understanding of the material presented in the outline is required to complete this activity.

2. Together with a student partner, use the panoramic procedure evaluation to assess your ability to satisfactorily perform each of the steps of the panoramic radiographic procedure.

   WARNING: **DO NOT ACTIVATE THE EXPOSURE BUTTON. DO NOT EXPOSE YOUR STUDENT PARTNER TO RADIATION. YOU ARE PRACTICING THESE SKILLS. YOU WILL NOT ACTUALLY EXPOSE THIS PRACTICE FILM.**

3. Instructor demonstration may enhance knowledge of the laboratory exercise.

4. Obtain instructor feedback on your performance as necessary or as instructed.

LABORATORY EXERCISE ACTIVITIES

Part 1: Cassette and Film Preparation

1. Obtain cassette with intensifying screens and a practice film.

2. Use Procedure 14.1 to practice cassette and film preparation.

3. Designate an area with counter space for this activity. Realistically this preparation step would be performed in the darkroom. However, practicing this step with the lights on may help you visual the skills you are developing.

Part 2: Unit Preparation

Together with a student partner, use Procedure 14.1 to prepare the panoramic radiographic unit. Follow infection control protocol for preparing the panoramic radiographic unit, and attach the loaded film cassette onto the unit.

Part 3: Patient Preparation

With your student partner playing the role of the patient, proceed with the steps outlined in Procedure 14.1 to prepare your patient for the panoramic radiograph.

Part 4: Patient Positioning

Position your student partner into the panoramic unit following the guidelines outlined in Procedure 14.1. Note that the patient must be positioned into all three dimensions of the focal trough.

Part 5: Exposure

1. Select appropriate exposure setting and simulate exposure.

   WARNING: **REMEMBER THAT YOU ARE PRACTICING PANORAMIC POSITIONING ONLY. DO NOT EXPOSE YOUR STUDENT PARTNER TO RADIATION.**

2. Utilize guidelines outlined in Procedure 14.1.

3. Release the patient.

4. Perform infection control protocol following the procedure.

COMPETENCY AND EVALUATION

1. Switch student partner roles and repeat this exercise. The student patient should now play the role of radiographer and the student radiographer should now play the role of patient, so that both partners have the opportunity to complete this exercise.

2. When both you and your partner have completed the exercise, each of you should review the panoramic procedure evaluation (Procedure 14.1) and determine what skills you found the most challenging and/or the easiest to learn.

   What steps do you anticipate being the easiest to master? Why?

   What steps do you anticipate being the most difficult to achieve? Why?

What are some examples of directions you had to give to the patient to achieve their cooperation with the procedure?

What visual guides did the manufacturer of the panoramic unit provide you for positioning the patient correctly? Explain how you used these guides to position the patient within the focal trough.

3. Complete the study questions.

Procedure 14.1

Panoramic Procedure Evaluation

Cassette and Film Preparation

1. Examine the cassette for proper function.   _____

   a. Examine the cassette for warping (rigid cassettes) or tears (plastic
      sleeve cassettes).   _____

   b. Check the hinge or Velcro^R seal for secure closing and a light-light
      seal. (Figure 11.6)   _____

2. Examine the intensifying screens for quality.   _____

   a. Check for scratches.   _____

   b. Check for need of cleaning.   _____

3. Ensure that the intensifying screens are properly secured to the cassette
   (rigid cassette) or are properly loaded into the flexible cassette. (Screens
   should be folded with the printed information identifying the screen
   manufacturer and screen type on the inside of the fold.) (See Figure 14.10)   _____

4. Obtain a box of panoramic film and place the film box and cassette with
   intensifying screens on darkroom counter. Turn off the white overhead
   light and turn on the safelight.   _____

5. Open the box of panoramic film, remove one sheet of panoramic film, and
   place in the cassette between the intensifying screens. Close the cassette and
   hinge to ensure a light-tight position. Resecure the panoramic film box and
   return to its storage place.   _____

*Satisfactorily
Performed*

Unit Preparation

1. Clean and disinfect with appropriate disinfectant all surfaces that will
   contact the patient either directly or indirectly. See the following list:

   a. Chin rest   _____

   b. Head positioner guides   _____

   c. Support handles   _____

   d. Chair or seat (sit down units only)   _____

   e. Lead (or lead-equivalent) apron   _____

(continued)

Procedure 14.1 *(continued)*

2. Select a sterile (disposable or autoclavable) bite guide. Load into the bite guide holder. (Use a sterile cotton roll to separate the arches if a bite guide is not used by the unit manufacturer.)

   _____

3. Attach the loaded film cassette to the panoramic x-ray unit according to the manufacturer's instructions. Align the cassette into proper position using guidelines established by manufacturer. (Figure 14.1 ■)

   _____

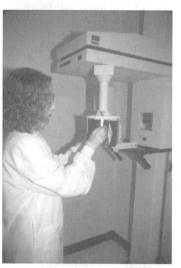

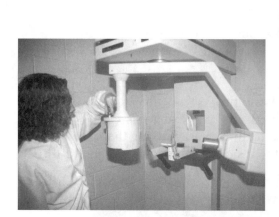

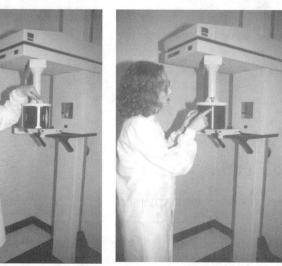

Figure 14.1 This manufacturer's recommendations for loading the cassette onto the panoramic unit include securing the lock pin to immobilize the cassette drum during attachment of the cassette, attaching the cassette to the drum with the arrow pointing toward the vertical column of the unit indicating correct alignment of the film on the rotating drum, unlocking the pin to allow the cassette drum to rotate throughout the exposure, and aligning the long white line of the cassette with the red line etched on the cassette drum to position the film at the beginning for exposure.

(continued)

Procedure 14.1 (continued)

Patient Preparation

1. Assess the patient for need of panoramic survey. _____

2. Inform the patient of the need for the radiograph, explain the procedure and rationale, answer patient concerns/questions regarding the radiographic procedure, and obtain the patient's written consent. _____

3. Request that the patient remove eyeglasses, necklaces, hair barrettes, facial jewelry (tongue, lip piercing adornments), removable dental appliances, and any other material that may interfere with the radiographic procedure such as chewing gum or a jacket with thickly padded shoulders. _____

4. Place the lead (or lead-equivalent) apron without a lead thyroid collar over the patient. (Figure 14.2 ■) _____

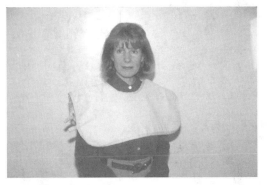

Figure 14.2 Lead barrier without the thyroid collar, appropriate for protecting the patient from scatter radiation exposure during the panoramic procedure.

Satisfactorily Performed

Patient Positioning

1. To position the patient into the focal trough's anterior/posterior dimension, instruct him/her to bite on the bite guide with the anterior teeth occluding edge-to-edge, or to place the chin completely forward into the chin rest or against the forehead rest. (Figure 14.3 ■) _____

2. To position the patient into the focal trough's lateral (right/left) dimension, close the head positioner guides or instruct the patient to view his/her reflection in the mirror (if available) and align the mid-saggital plane perpendicular to the floor. (Figure 14.4 ■) Use the panoramic machine's indictor light, if so equipped, to locate the mid-sagittal place. _____

(continued)

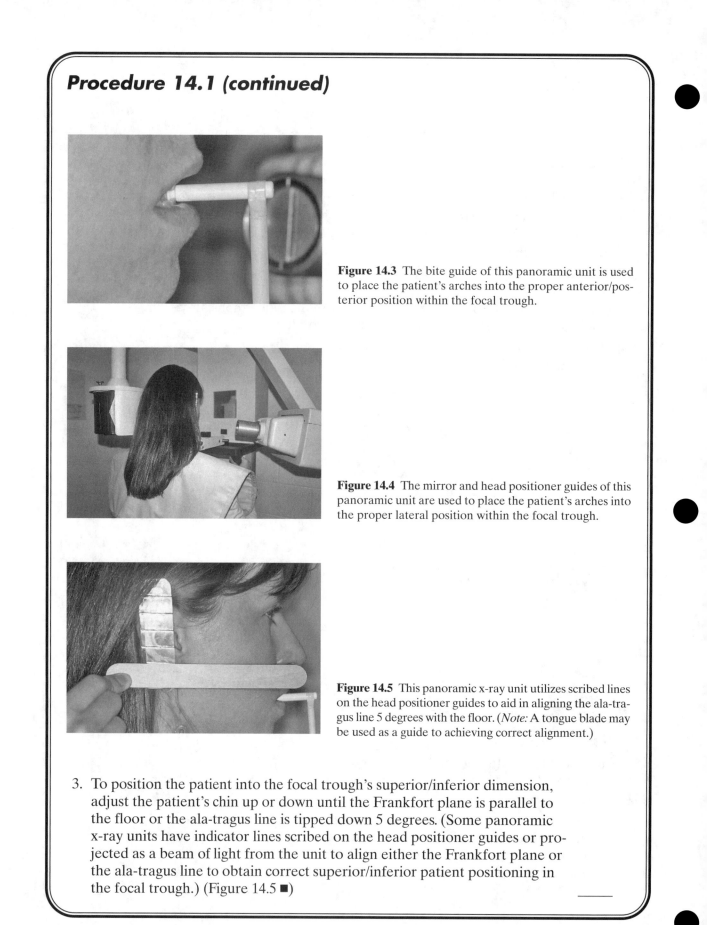

Figure 14.3 The bite guide of this panoramic unit is used to place the patient's arches into the proper anterior/posterior position within the focal trough.

Figure 14.4 The mirror and head positioner guides of this panoramic unit are used to place the patient's arches into the proper lateral position within the focal trough.

Figure 14.5 This panoramic x-ray unit utilizes scribed lines on the head positioner guides to aid in aligning the ala-tragus line 5 degrees with the floor. (*Note:* A tongue blade may be used as a guide to achieving correct alignment.)

3. To position the patient into the focal trough's superior/inferior dimension, adjust the patient's chin up or down until the Frankfort plane is parallel to the floor or the ala-tragus line is tipped down 5 degrees. (Some panoramic x-ray units have indicator lines scribed on the head positioner guides or projected as a beam of light from the unit to align either the Frankfort plane or the ala-tragus line to obtain correct superior/inferior patient positioning in the focal trough.) (Figure 14.5 ■)

(continued)

Procedure 14.1 (continued)

Exposure

1. Select the appropriate kVp and mA for this patient. Refer to posted exposure settings. The exposure time setting is preset by the manufacturer. _____

2. Instruct the patient to swallow and place the tongue up against the hard palate and to close his/her lips around the bite guide or cotton roll. _____

3. Instruct the patient to remain still throughout the exposure cycle. _____

4. Take an appropriate position where you are protected from radiation exposure, and simulate depressing the exposure button for the duration of the cycle. _____

5. Release the patient. Discard the disposable bite guide or, if autoclavable, prepare for sterilization. Clean and disinfect with appropriate disinfectant all surfaces that came in contact either directly or indirectly with the patient. See the following list: _____

   a. Chin rest _____

   b. Head positioner guides _____

   c. Support handles _____

   d. Chair or seat (sit down units only) _____

   e. Lead (or lead-equivalent) apron _____

*Satisfactorily
Performed*

Processing

1. Remove the film cassette with film from the panoramic unit, and return to the darkroom. Turn off the overhead white light, and turn on the safe light. _____

2. Open the cassette and carefully remove the film. Handle with clean dry, ungloved hands. Load the film into the automatic processor or the manual film processing rack for processing. _____

3. Label the processed film with the patient's name, date, and other pertinent information. _____

NOTE: If using radiographic tape for identification, attach the label to the front of cassette prior to exposing the film. If using a commercial flash identification printer, fill out a flash printer card and flash print after the exposure, but prior to processing the film. (Figure 14.8 and Figure 14.9)

I. Panoramic radiographs
   A. Uses
      1. Detection of large lesions
      2. Evaluation of unexplained asymmetry
      3. Assess growth and development
      4. Assess the need for orthodontic intervention
      5. Detection of fractures in supporting bone
      6. Evaluation of third molar impactions
      7. Assessment of condition of underlying bone prior to implants or denture construction
   B. Advantages over intraoral radiographs
      1. Increased coverage of supporting structures of the oral cavity.
      2. Reduced patient radiation dose over an intraoral full mouth series of radiographs.
      3. Can be performed in less time than the exposure of a full mouth series of radiographs.
      4. Simple procedure to perform.
      5. Minimal patient discomfort.
      6. May be performed on patients who cannot tolerate placement of an intraoral film packet.
      7. Requires minimal patient instruction and cooperation.
      8. Infection control protocol minimized.
      9. Panoramic broad-view image of the entire arches is easy for patients to understand when utilizing for patient education and in explaining treatment plans.
   C. Limitations
      1. Increased image distortion.
      2. Reduced image sharpness.
      3. Focal trough size and shape limits imagery to only those structures that fit into the image layer.
      4. Soft tissue shadows and ghost images present on the resulting image may hinder interpretation.
      5. Not useful in detecting incipient carious lesions or early periodontal changes.
      6. Simple procedure may cause the panoramic radiograph to be overused inappropriately as a screening film.
      7. Length of exposure time may limit its use on young children and other patients who cannot remain still throughout the exposure cycle.
      8. Cost of a panoramic unit may be a significant burden on the practice.
   D. Equipment
      1. Rotational x-ray tube head
         a. Fixed vertical angulation of the PID at approximately negative 8 degrees.
         b. Collimation of the PID produces a narrow, fan shaped x-ray beam.

2. Cassette holder (drum)
   a. The cassette with intensifying screens attaches to the cassette holder (drum).
   b. Moves the film at the same speed as the rotational beam.
3. Patient positioning guides
   a. Anterior/posterior position is determined through the use of a bite guide, forehead rest, or anterior edge of the chin rest.
   b. Lateral (right/left) position is determined through the use of side head positioner guides, a mirror, or beams of light that shine on the patient's face to assist with determining the position of the mid-saggital plane.
   c. Superior/inferior position is determined through the use of a chin rest or beams of light that shine on the patient's face to assist with determining the position of the Frankfort plane or ala-tragus line.
4. Exposure control panel
   a. Variable kVp
     1) Setting is recommended by manufacturer.
     2) Usually based on the size and density of the patient and the area to be imaged.
   b. Variable or fixed mA
   c. Fixed exposure time
     1) Preset by the manufacturer
     2) Approximately 15–20 seconds to complete the exposure cycle

E. Technique
1. Tomography
   a. "Slice" or "layer" of tissue imaged
   b. Several different x-ray beam movement patterns are utilized to produce an image.
   c. Each section of the simultaneously moving film is exposed until the entire image is complete.
2. Focal trough
   a. Horseshoe-shaped area corresponding to the shape of the average dental arches.
     1) Focal trough size and shape is determined by the manufacturer.
     2) Average dimensions do not always accommodate every patient.
   b. Objects located in the focal trough will be imaged in acceptable detail on the resultant radiograph.
   c. Objects located outside the focal trough will be blurred out of focus on the resultant radiograph.
     1) As ghost images that may compromise image clarity.
     2) Objects positioned outside the focal trough may not be detected.

II. Panoramic procedure
A. Cassette and film preparation
1. Inspect cassettes for wear.
2. Check hinges for proper light tight seals. (See Figure 11.6)

3. Handle intensifying screens with care.
   a. Do not touch screens with fingers.
   b. Clean only as necessary and as recommended by manufacturer. (Aggressive cleaning can damage screens.)
   c. Apply a manufacturer recommended antistatic solution as necessary.
4. Select panoramic film to match the intensifying screens.
   a. Rare earth intensifying screens
      1) Fluoresce green light.
      2) Use extraoral film that is sensitive to green light.
   b. Calcium tungstate intensifying screens
      1) Fluoresce blue light.
      2) Use extraoral film that is sensitive to blue light.

B. Unit preparation
   1. Infection control protocol is less complicated than intraoral radiography.
      a. All parts of the unit that contact or will have the potential to contact the patient must be cleaned and disinfected.
      b. Disposable plastic barriers may be indicated. (Figure 14.6 ■).
      c. Bite guide must be sterilized if disposable bite guides are not available.
   2. Loaded film cassette should be attached to the cassette holder (drum).
      a. Cassette must be attached according to manufacturer's recommendations, so that the film will be aligned to move in the appropriate direction once the cycle begins.
      b. Cassette must be attached according to manufacturer's recommendations, so that the exposure will begin at the beginning edge of film.

C. Patient preparation
   1. Explain the procedure to the patient.
   2. Request that the patient remove all metal or dense objects that may be in the path of the primary beam (eyeglasses, necklaces,

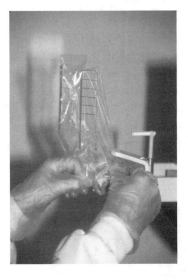

Figure 14.6 Plastic barriers may be placed over the chin rest, head positioner guides, and other parts of the panoramic unit that contact the patient.

hair barrettes, facial jewelry [tongue, lip piercing adornments], removable dental appliances).

     3. Coats and jackets with thickly padded shoulders may interfere with the rotation of the cassette drum or the tube head and should be removed.

     4. Request that the patient remain still throughout the exposure cycle.

D. Patient positioning

     1. Follow manufacturer's recommendations for placing the patient into the focal trough.

       a. In the anterior/posterior dimension

       b. In the lateral (right/left) dimension

       c. In the superior/inferior dimension

     2. Request that the patient close lips around the bite guide or a cotton roll to prevent imaging the soft tissue shadow of the lip line.

     3. Request that the patient swallow and place the tongue against the roof of the mouth throughout the exposure cycle to fill in the oral cavity and to minimize the appearance of a large radiolucent image of an open air space.

E. Exposure selection

     1. kVp

       a. Controls the penetrating ability of the x-ray beam.

       b. Set according to manufacturer's recommendations.

         1) Based on size and density of the patient and the area being imaged.

         2) Higher kVp setting required for increased size and density.

         3) Lower kVp setting required for decreased size and density.

     2. mA

       a. Controls the amount of radiation.

       b. Set according to manufacturer's recommendations.

     3. Exposure time

       a. Exposure time is not variable for panoramic exposures.

       b. Exposure time is preset by manufacturer.

F. Processing

     1. Process according to manufacturer's recommendations.

     2. Panoramic films may be processed automatically or manually.

G. Labeling

     1. Most panoramic units have a method of indicating left and right sides of the radiograph. (Figure 14.7 ■)

     2. If the panoramic unit does not have a built-in method of labeling the right and left sides of the radiograph, a lead letter may be affixed to the cassette prior to exposing.

     3. Radiographic tape is also available to label panoramic films. The patient's name and other identifying characteristics may also be permanently recorded onto the image with radiographic tape. (Figure 14.8 ■)

     4. A commercial flash printer unit may be used to permanently record pertinent information onto the patient's radiograph. (Figure 14.9 ■)

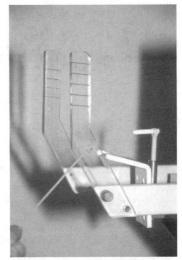

Figure 14.7 A lead letter is used by this panoramic unit to identify the right side of the patient's radiograph.

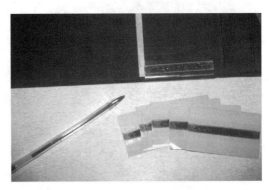

Figure 14.8 Radiographic tape may be used to identify a patient's panoramic radiograph.

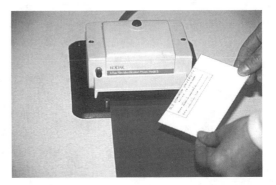

Figure 14.9 A flash printer may be used to identify a patient's radiographic film.

III. Panoramic radiographic errors
    A. Cassette and film preparation
        1. Errors
            a. Cassette not closed light tight
            b. Film not seated at the fold of (flexible plastic-sleeve) cassette
            c. Intensifying screens placed into the cassette inside out (with manufacturer's labeling on the outside) (Figure 14.10 ■)
            d. Film not placed in between the intensifying screens (flexible plastic-sleeve cassette)
            e. Mistaken use of duplicating film instead of panoramic film (Figure 14.11 ■)

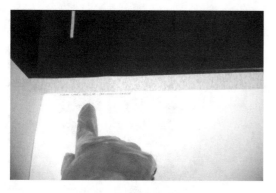

Figure 14.10 The side of the intensifying screens with the manufacturer's labeling should be facing the film.

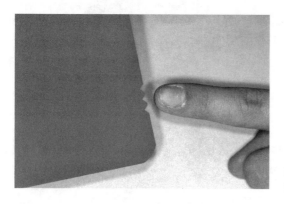

Figure 14.11 Duplicating film is distinguished from panoramic film by the notched edge placed by the manufacturer.

     f. Intensifying screens scratched or damaged

     g. Double exposure

  2. Evidenced by

     a. Increased density from accidental light exposure

     b. A portion of the film not exposed (blank/clear)

     c. A blank/clear or very light image where intensifying screens were reversed

     d. A blank/clear or very light image when film was placed outside the intensifying screens

     e. A blank/clear film when duplicating film is mistakenly used

     f. A radiopaque artifact corresponding to the damaged screen area

     g. Dark image of two separate exposures superimposed on top of each other that is confusing to interpret

B. Unit preparation

  1. Errors

     a. Film cassette drum not set to rotate freely throughout the exposure

     b. Film cassette not correctly aligned to begin exposure at the beginning of the cycle

  2. Evidenced by

     a. A blank/clear image with a dense vertical band of overexposure, representing the only area of the film to be exposed

     b. A generally blank/clear image with a narrow band of exposure at one end, representing where the film then proceeded to rotate in the opposite direction of the radiation source

C. Patient preparation
1. Errors
   a. Tube head or cassette holder (drum) contacted the patient's shoulder during rotation.
   b. Patient wore a metal or dense object that was in the path of the primary beam during exposure.
   c. A lead thyroid collar was used during the exposure.
2. Evidenced by
   a. Radiolucent vertical band(s) of overexposure in the areas where the unit was stopped temporarily, overexposing certain regions of the film
   b. Radiopaque artifacts from the object left in the path of the x-ray beam; artifacts of the object's ghost image evident
   c. An unexposed area, usually located at the inferior edge of the film
D. Patient positioning
1. Errors
   a. Arches not positioned in the anterior/posterior dimension of the focal trough.
   b. Arches not positioned in the lateral (right/left) dimension of the focal trough.
   c. Arches not positioned in the superior/inferior dimension of the focal trough.
   d. Patient not standing/sitting up straight.
   e. Patient's head is tilted.
2. Evidenced by
   a. Anterior teeth which are diminished in size indicate the arches were positioned too far anteriorly in the focal trough.
   b. Anterior teeth which are magnified in size indicate that the arches were positioned too far posteriorly in the focal trough.
   c. Posterior teeth which are diminished in size on the right side and magnified in size on the left side indicate that the arches were positioned too far to the right in the focal trough.
   d. Posterior teeth which are magnified in size on the right side and diminished in size on the left side indicate that the arches were positioned too far to the left in the focal trough.
   e. An exaggerated "frown" appearance to the overall image indicates the arches were positioned too far superiorly in the focal trough (chin up).
   f. An exaggerated "smile" appearance to the overall image indicates the arches were positioned too far inferiorly in the focal trough (chin down).
   g. Radiopaque ghost image of the spinal column usually superimposed over the mandibular anterior teeth.
   h. Image appears tilted.
E. Exposure
1. Errors
   a. Incorrect exposure setting selected.
   b. Patient not instructed to close lips around bite guide or cotton roll.

c. Bite guide or cotton roll not utilized to separate the arches.

d. Patient not instructed to place tongue against palate during exposure.

e. Patient moved during the procedure.

2. Evidenced by

a. An over/underexposed image.

b. An image of the soft tissue shadow of the lip line across the anterior teeth resembling a fracture.

c. Incisal/occlusal edges of the maxillary and mandibular teeth superimposed on top of each other.

d. A large radiolucency in the apex area of the maxillary teeth.

e. A blurred portion or irregular margins of the image.

F. Processing

1. Errors

a. Over/underdeveloped

b. Static electricity artifacts

c. Glove powder artifacts

2. Evidenced by

a. An image that is too dark/light

b. Radiolucent lines, spots, or smudges indicating white light exposure from the static charge

c. Radiolucent powder smudges

BIBLIOGRAPHY

Haring, JI, Howerton, LJ. *Dental Radiography. Principles and Techniques,* 3rd ed. St. Louis, MO: Elsevier; 2006: 310–317.

Eastman Kodak Company. *Successful Panoramic Radiography.* Rochester, NY: Eastman Kodak Company; 2000.

Whaites, E. *Essentials of Dental Radiography and Radiology,* 3rd ed. New York, NY: Churchill Livingstone; 2002.

1. All of the following are indications for exposing a panoramic radiograph *except* one. Which one is this *exception?*
    A. Caries detection
    B. Location of an impaction
    C. Evaluation of eruption patterns
    D. Imaging a large lesion

2. Which of the following terms refers to the horseshoe-shaped zone of sharpness where an object would be imaged in acceptable detail?
    A. Cassette drum
    B. Ghost image
    C. Intensifying screen
    D. Focal trough

3. When a patient's arches are positioned too far to the right, the teeth on the _____ side of the image will appear magnified.
    A. right
    B. left

4. When a patient's arches are positioned too far to the left, the teeth on the _____ side of the image will appear magnified.
    A. right
    B. left

5. When a patient's anterior teeth are positioned too far forward in the focal trough (closer to the film), the anterior teeth will be _____ in size.
    A. magnified
    B. diminished

6. When a patient's anterior teeth are positioned too far back in the focal trough (closer to the PID), the anterior teeth will be _____ in size.
    A. magnified
    B. diminished

7. When a patient's chin is tipped too far upward, the resulting radiograph image will appear to
    A. frown
    B. smile

8. When a patient's chin is tipped too far downward, the resulting radiograph image will appear to
    A. frown
    B. smile

9. A dark shadow obscuring the apices of the maxillary anterior teeth is most likely caused by which of the following?
    A. Lead apron got in the way
    B. Facial jewelry not removed
    C. Chin not rested on chin rest
    D. Tongue not resting against palate
    E. Patient not occluded on bite guide/cotton roll

10. A patient who wears a maxillary full denture needs a panoramic radiograph. All of his natural mandibular teeth in place. You will request that the patient remove the denture during the exposure. What patient positioning step do you anticipate having the most difficulty achieving? If an error is made in this step, how will the resultant image look? Why? What corrective actions would you take? Why?

_____

_____

_____

_____

_____

_____

_____

_____

_____

_____

laboratory exercise 15

Digital Radiography

INTRODUCTION

Technological advancements in health care have prompted dentistry to embrace the possibility of improving the quality of oral health care through the use of digital radiography. Many practices have already made the transition from film-based radiography to digital imaging. (Figure 15.1 ■) Others are beginning to incorporate digital radiography into their practices. Today's dental assisting and dental hygiene students are sure to encounter digital radiography during their careers.

The purpose of this laboratory exercise is to introduce the student to one type of digital imaging system. While there are numerous digital imaging systems on the market, experience operating the computer, positioning the sensor, viewing radiographic images on a monitor, and utilizing software to manipulate the images will help introduce the student this technology.

OBJECTIVES

Following completion of this lab activity, you will be able to:

1. Identify the components of a digital imaging system.

2. Place and expose a digital sensor to produce a diagnostic quality image.

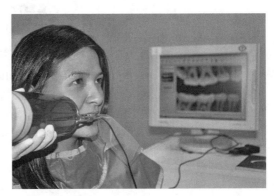

Figure 15.1 Radiographic procedure using digital imagery.

3. Maintain infection control during the radiographic procedure using a digital imaging system.

4. Demonstrate examples of digital image manipulation that will enhance the diagnostic quality of a digital radiograph.

MATERIALS

Teaching manikin or skull

Lead (or lead-equivalent) apron with thyroid collar

Digital imaging system with bitewing sensor

Bitewing sensor-holding device (recommended by the manufacturer of the digital imaging system)

Infection control barriers (recommended by the manufacturer of the digital imaging system)

Printer

PREPARATION

1. Study the chapter outline to prepare for this laboratory exercise. An understanding of the material presented in the outline is required to complete this activity.

2. Utilize Procedure 15.1 to assist you with completing the exercises. Your instructor may perform a demonstration to familiarize you with the digital system at your facility.

3. Prepare radiology operatory. Set up teaching manikin or skull. Ensure that correct "patient" positioning is achieved. Ensure that the occlusal plane is parallel to the floor and the midsagittal plane is perpendicular to the floor.

4. Place lead apron (or lead-equivalent barrier) and thyroid collar over the "patient."

5. Obtain instructor feedback on your performance as necessary or as instructed.

LABORATORY EXERCISE ACTIVITIES

Part 1: Horizontal Bitewings Using the Digital Imaging System-Technique

1. Prepare the sensor for placement intraorally. (Figure 15.2 ■)

2. Attach the sensor to the bitewing holder. (Figure 15.3 ■)

3. Check posted exposure settings for the dental x-ray unit, and set for digital bitewing radiographs. See the manufacturer's recommendations for what settings to use with the digital system at your facility. Many digital sensors require 50 percent less radiation than that required for "F" speed film.

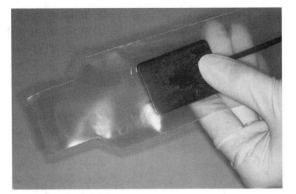

Figure 15.2 Wired digital sensor being covered with a plastic barrier.

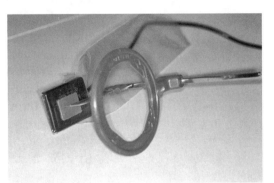

Figure 15.3 A wired sensor attached to a film holder, ready for positioning intraorally.

4. Place and expose the series of bitewing radiographs in the following order:

1st   right premolar bitewing

2nd   right molar bitewing

3rd   left premolar bitewing

4th   left molar bitewing

Note: Left-handed radiographers may use this order:

1st   left premolar bitewing

2nd   left molar bitewing

3rd   right premolar bitewing

4th   right molar bitewing

Part 2: Interpretation of Digital Images

1. Evaluate the images.

2. Print the set of bitewing images to a hard copy. Do not close the file.

3. Next, using the computer software change the following:
   a. Right molar bitewing—increase the density
   b. Right premolar bitewing—increase the contrast
   c. Left premolar bitewing—enlarge the image (magnification tool)

d. Left molar bitewing—manipulate the image using one of the software tools such as reversing the gray scale, embossing, colorization, and so on

4. Print the set of bitewing images that have been manipulated.

COMPETENCY AND EVALUATION

1. Obtain instructor feedback. Identify which step (packet placement, vertical angulation, horizontal angulation, centering) needs improvement.

2. Repeat Part 1 and Part 2 at the direction of your instructor.

3. Examine the first printout of your digital images. Evaluate your technique. Are the radiographic images diagnostic? Were you able to transfer the skills you learned with film-based radiography to this technology? What did you discover to be the most challenging aspect of digital radiographic technology? What is your opinion of this technology? Do you prefer one, digital imaging or film-based radiography, over the other? Why? Which do you think patients will prefer? What advantages and disadvantages did you encounter using this technology for this exercise?

4. Examine the second printout of your digital images. What are the advantages and disadvantages of the software tools utilized for this exercise? Did the system mark the second printout as a manipulated image? What might be the legal ramifications of digital imagery?

5. Complete the study questions.

Procedure Box 15.1

Digital Radiographic Procedure

1. Activate computer exam window.
   a. Turn on the computer.
   b. Open the digital imaging system program from the desktop window.
   c. Chose "new exam" from the task bar.
   d. Type your name (*last & first*) into the patient name box.
   e. Choose the four horizontal bitewings window.
   f. Highlight the box representing the first exposure. (Figure 15.4 ■)

2. Prepare sensor for placement intraorally.
   a. Wipe the sensor with an appropriate disinfectant recommended by the manufacturer. Many sensors can be wiped with an intermediate-level disinfectant. Place the plastic sheath recommended by the manufacturer over the sensor. Use only FDA-cleared disposable plastic barriers.
   b. Chose the appropriate film holder recommended by the manufacturer and place on the sensor over the plastic sheath. (Figure 15.3)

3. Turn on the x-ray unit and adjust exposure settings.
   a. See the manufacturer's recommendation. Exposure time may possibly be reduced to one-half the time required for "F" speed film.

4. Place the sensor intraorally.
   a. Ensure that you place the sensor into the position you selected when you highlighted the film box in Step 1.f (Figure 15.4)

5. Activate the exposure button.
   a. Wait for the image to appear on the computer monitor.

6. Evaluate the image.
   a. Do not remove the sensor from the patient's mouth yet. First, follow your digital software program instructions to zoom in on the image and evaluate. If you need to retake the exposure, simply adjust the sensor placement to correct the error noted without completely removing it from the patient's mouth.
   b. After repositioning the sensor, follow your digital software program instructions to retake the image and activate the re-exposure.

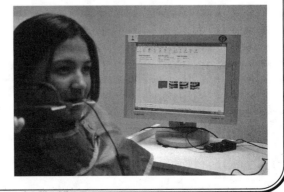

Figure 15.4 Highlighted box indicating that the radiographer is ready to position the patient's right molar bitewing radiograph.

I. Film-less radiographic images
   A. Digital versus analog (Figure 15.5 ■)
      1. Black-and-white film-based radiographs are considered analog because the distribution of the silver halide crystals create a continuous density pattern
      2. Digital refers to a numeric format of the image; distinct pixels (picture elements) create the image
      3. Digital images have no physical form but exist as bits of information in a computer file
   B. Process (Figure 15.1)
      1. Image is captured on a sensor.
      2. An electronic charge is produced on the surface of the sensor.
      3. The digitized signal is transmitted to a computer.
      4. The computer processes the signal and produces an image on a monitor.

II. Equipment
   A. An x-ray machine
      1. Conventional x-ray machine may be used for both film-based and digital radiography.
      2. 70 kVp or less is ideal for producing digital radiographs.
      3. Low milliamperage, 5 mA or less, is ideal for producing digital radiographs.
      4. Timer may have to be adjusted so that it is capable of generating a low radiation dose output.
   B. Sensor
      1. Replaces film
      2. May be wired to the computer or wireless, sending the information to the computer via radio frequency
      3. Available in different sizes
      4. Types
         a. Charge-coupled device (CCD)
            1) Most common type of sensor used for dental digital radiography.
            2) Introduced to dental digital radiography in 1987.
            3) Thin wafer of silicon that contains an electronic circuit.

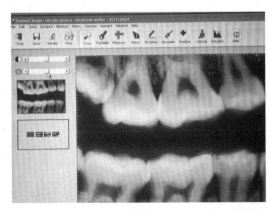

Figure 15.5 Example of a digital radiographic image. Note that the image contrast and density may be adjusted utilizing the computer software.

4) The circuit contains individual pixels arranged in a matrix (the pixels are the silver halide equivalent of film).
5) Radiation is deposited into each pixel "well" within the matrix creating the latent image.
6) The latent image is then transferred to the computer via a wire or via radio frequency.
b. Complementary metal oxide semiconductor (CMOS)
   1) Typically found in video cameras.
   2) Currently only two companies utilize CMOS technology for dental digital radiographic systems.
   3) Like CCD, CMOS technology uses a silicon chip, but is less expense to produce.
   4) The difference between CCD and CMOS technology is in the way the pixel charges are read by the computer.
   5) In CMOS technology, pixels are isolated from one another and connected separately and directly to a transmitter that stores and displays the energy as a digital gray value.
c. Photo-stimulable phosphor (PSP)
   1) Phosphor-coated plates absorb and store x-rays.
   2) The energy stored is later released as light (phosphorescence) when stimulated with a laser device.
   3) PSP plates are not wired to the computer.
   4) Plates are exposed and then placed into a laser device that converts the stored energy to an image.
   5) The plates must be erased by exposing them to a bright light source prior to reusing.
   6) Utilizing a laser device to process the plates is the equivalent step to darkroom processing film-based radiographs.
C. Computer
   1. Responsible for converting the energy stored in the sensor into an image that can be read off a monitor.
   2. Images are usually available for viewing on the computer monitor within 0.5 to 120 seconds following exposure.
   3. Computer should provide adequate storage of radiographic image files.
   4. An Internet connection allows for electronic transfer of images between practices for consultations and referrals or to third-party payment providers for approval of treatment.
D. Software
   1. Provides variations in viewing the images
   2. Ability to view images side-be-side; enlarged or magnified; multiple images on one screen.
   3. Features that allow the radiographer to manipulate the image to improve the density or contrast (Figure 15.5).
   4. Many digital software manufacturers provide software features such as reversing the gray scale, embossing, colorization, to change the way the image appears on the screen as an aid in diagnosis (Figure 15.6 ■).

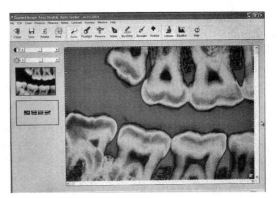

Figure 15.6 The use of software allows manipulation of the image.

5. Quality software programs imprint manipulated images with an identification that labels the image as changed from the original.
6. Digital subtraction
   a. Process by which two images acquired at different points in treatment may be superimposed on each other.
   b. Unchanged anatomy will cancel each other out of the image, whereas changes will appear distinctly imaged.
   c. Valuable in assessing bone loss or regeneration.
   d. Digital subtraction requires the use of standard sensor placement and precise x-ray beam angulations.
III. Methods of acquiring a digital image
   A. Indirect
      1. A scanner is used to convert film-based radiographs into digital images.
      2. Uses a special transparency device attached to flat bed scanner.
      3. Digital photography may be used to take a digital image of a film-based radiograph.
   B. Direct
      1. Uses a digital sensor to capture the image.
      2. The digital sensor transmits the signal received from the exposure to the computer via a wire attachment or radio frequency.
IV. Characteristics of a digital image
   A. Contrast resolution
      1. Contrast allows the viewer to distinguish between different densities (light or dark areas) on the image.
      2. Dental digital sensors are capable of capturing 256 to over 65,000 different densities.
      3. Computer monitors reserve the use of some gray levels for their operating system, so most computer monitors currently available only display about 242 levels of gray.
      4. The human eye is capable of detecting about 30 levels of gray.
      5. Due to its ability to record many levels of gray and increase contrast resolution, there is potential for the computer to aid in diagnosis; however, current software programs are not able to do this better than the human practitioner.

B. Spatial resolution
   1. Defined as the ability to distinguish between closely spaced objects.
   2. The number and size of the pixels determines spatial resolution.
   3. Less pixels produce an image with jagged edges; more pixels produce a smoother image.
   4. Spatial resolution is often measured in line pairs per millimeter (lp/mm).
      a. Defined as the ability to distinguished between very fine sets of radiopaque lines.
      b. The greater the spatial resolution the sharper the image.
      c. The unaided human eye can distinguish between approximately 60 lp/mm.
      d. Film-based radiographs record approximately 200 lp/mm.
      e. Digital images displayed on a computer monitor reveal approximately 70 lp/mm.
      f. When software is utilized to magnify a digital image, the image begins to look jagged and take on a "building block" appearance, indicating the limited spatial resolution obtained with digital radiography.
C. Digital sensor sensitivity to radiation
   1. Digital sensors are more sensitive to radiation exposure than film.
   2. Depending on the manufacturer, digital sensors may require as little as 50 to 80% less radiation than film-based radiography.
   3. Currently there is no rating system to classify the speed of digital sensors; information on the reduction in radiation exposure with the use of digital sensors is based on manufacturers' claims.
V. Advantages and disadvantages of digital imaging compared with film-based radiography
   A. Advantages
      1. Less radiation dose to the patient.
      2. Instant viewing of the image.
      3. Saves time.
      4. Eliminates the need for darkroom, chemicals, generation of hazardous wastes.
      5. Potential to improve the image without reexposing the patient (density and contrast may be improved through the use of software).
      6. Improved gray scale has the potential to aid in diagnosis.
      7. Electronic transfer of images via the Internet speeds communication between professionals and third-party payment providers.
      8. Enhanced patient education, utilizing the computer monitor to view the images.
   B. Disadvantages
      1. Initial investment costs.
      2. Timing of when to purchase the system; as technology advances, equipment changes may make equipment obsolete in a relatively short time.

3. Reliability of computer stored patient records; the possibility of malfunction and record loss is enormous.
4. System compatibility with other professionals, third-party providers, and to equipment updates in the future.
5. Time and efforts required to learn the system and transfer technique and interpretative skills from film-based radiography to digital imaging.
6. Sensor size and bulk may make ideal intraoral placement on some patients difficult.
7. Wired sensors may be difficult to position intraorally.
8. Sensors require careful infection control based on the manufacturer's precise recommendations; sensors cannot be heat sterilized; protective plastic barriers have been known to tear and expose the sensor to the oral cavity.
9. Legal concerns with images that may have been altered through software manipulation.

BIBLIOGRAPHY

Haring, JI, Howerton, LJ. *Dental Radiography. Principles and Techniques,* 3rd ed. St. Louis, MO: Elsevier; 2006: 343–354.

Johnson, ON, Thomson, EM. *Essentials of Dental Radiography for Dental Assistants and Hygienists,* 8th ed. Upper Saddle River, NJ: Prentice Hall; 2007: 349–365.

Mauriello, SM, Platin, E. Dental digital radiographic imaging. *Journal of Dental Hygiene.* 2001; 75:323–331.

Palenik, CJ. Infection control for dental radiography. *Dentistry Today.* 2004; 23:52–55.

White, SC, Pharoah, MJ. *Oral Radiology Principles and Interpretation,* 5th ed. St. Louis, MO: Elsevier; 2004: 225–244.

1. Distinct pixels, arranged numerically to form a radiographic image, are referred to as a (an)
   - A. Analog image
   - B. Digital image
   - C. Latent image
   - D. Film-based image

2. A _____ is used to capture an image by sending a digitized signal to a computer for viewing on a monitor.
   - A. Software program
   - B. Radio frequency
   - C. Scanner
   - D. Sensor

3. All of the following are necessary to produce a digital radiograph *except* one. Which one is this *exception?*
   - A. Computer
   - B. Sensor
   - C. Film
   - D. X-ray machine
   - E. Special software

4. Which of the following is considered ideal for producing digital images?
   - A. 70 kVp, 15 mA
   - B. 70 kVp, 5 mA
   - C. 90 kVp, 15 mA
   - D. 90 kVp, 5 mA

5. Which of the following types of sensors requires a "processing" step where the sensor must be read using a laser device?
   - A. CCD
   - B. CMOS
   - C. PSP

6. All of the following may be necessary to indirectly produce a digital image *except* one. Which one is this *exception?*
   - A. Sensor
   - B. Scanner
   - C. Digital camera
   - D. Computer
   - E. Film-based radiograph

7. Which of the following terms is defined as the ability to distinguish between closely spaced objects.
   - A. Contrast
   - B. Density
   - C. Spatial resolution
   - D. Sensitivity
   - E. Gray level

8. All of the following are considered advantages of digital imaging when compared with film-based imaging *except* one. Which one is this *exception?*

    A. Less radiation required.

    B. Less time required to produce an image.

    C. Darkroom can be updated to a digital darkroom.

    D. Electronic transfer of images speeds consultations.

    E. Image contrast and density can be improved without reexposing the patient.

9. All of the following are considered disadvantages of digital imaging when compared with film-based imaging *except* one. Which one is this *exception?*

    A. Initial investment costs.

    B. Images contain more gray shade levels.

    C. Technological compatibility with other systems.

    D. Images have the potential to be legally less reliable.

    E. Sensor size may be less tolerated than a film packet.

10. Which of the following infecton control methods is required for intraoral digital sensors?

    A. Disinfect and cover with a plastic barrier.

    B. Ultrasonic with detergent and dry heat sterilize.

    C. Wash with soap and water and cover with a plastic barrier.

    D. Disinfect and autoclave (moist heat under pressure).

    E. Wash with soap and water, ultrasonic with detergent, autoclave sterilize, and then cover with a plastic barrier just prior to use.

Answers to Study Questions

LABORATORY EXERCISE 1
Radiographic Film Processing and Darkroom Design and Maintenance

1.	A	4.	B	7.	B
2.	C	5.	C	8.	A
3.	D	6.	A	9.	B

10. Essay—See outline for key points to be included in this answer.

LABORATORY EXERCISE 2
Bitewing Radiographic Technique

1.	C	5.	A	9.	B
2.	C	6.	C	10.	D
3.	D	7.	D		
4.	B	8.	C		

LABORATORY EXERCISE 3
Periapical Radiographs—Paralleling Technique

1.	C	5.	B	9.	B
2.	B	6.	A	10.	C
3.	C	7.	A		
4.	D	8.	B		

LABORATORY EXERCISE 4
Periapical Radiographs—Bisecting Technique

1.	B	4.	A	7.	B
2.	D	5.	B	8.	B
3.	A	6.	B	9.	C

10. Essay—See outline for key points in Chapters 3 and 4 to be included in this answer.

LABORATORY EXERCISE 5
Radiographic Techniques with Supplemental Film Holders

1. B
2. C
3. A
4. C
5. C
6. E
7. Matching: A; B; A; A; B; A;B
8. A

9. Essay—See outline for key points to be included in this answer.

10. (c, f) The instrument assembly pictured on the top left is used to place periapical films intraorally to image the patient's maxillary right and mandibular left posterior regions. (d, e) The instrument assembly pictured on the top right is used to place periapical films intraorally to image the patient's maxillary left and mandibular right posterior regions. (b) The instrument assembly pictured on the bottom left is used to place periapical films intraorally to image the patient's maxillary and mandibular anterior regions. (a) The instrument assembly pictured on the bottom right is used to place bite-wing films intraorally to image the patient's anterior and posterior regions.

LABORATORY EXERCISE 6
Infection Control and Student Partner Practice

1. A
2. B
3. C
4. D
5. D
6. B
7. B
8. A
9. D

10. Essay—See outline for key points to be included in this answer.

LABORATORY EXERCISE 7
Patient Management and Student Partner Practice

1. D
2. C
3. A
4. B
5. B
6. C
7. B
8. D
9. A

10. Essay—Reflect on your laboratory experience to evaluate your progress.

LABORATORY EXERCISE 8
Film Mounting and Radiographic Landmarks

1. C
2. A
3. A
4. C
5. A
6. D
7. A
8. B
9. A
10. A.

LABORATORY EXERCISE 9
Exposure Variables—Factors Affecting the Radiographic Image

1. A	4. B	7. A
2. B	5. A	8. A
3. B	6. B	9. D

10.
$$\frac{100}{?} = \frac{8^2}{16^2} \qquad \frac{(4)100}{?} = \frac{1(4)}{4} \qquad\qquad \frac{12}{?} = \frac{8^2}{16^2} \qquad \frac{(4)12}{?} = \frac{1(4)}{4}$$

$$\frac{100}{?} = \frac{1^2}{2^2} \qquad \frac{(?)400}{?} = 1(?) \qquad\qquad \frac{12}{?} = \frac{1^2}{2^2} \qquad \frac{(?)48}{?} = 1(?)$$

$$\frac{100}{?} = \frac{1}{4} \qquad\quad 400 = ? \qquad\qquad\qquad \frac{12}{?} = \frac{1}{4} \qquad\quad 48 = ?$$

LABORATORY EXERCISE 10
Identifying and Correcting Radiographic Errors

1. E	4. B	7. A
2. C	5. A	8. A
3. A	6. E	9. B

10. Essay—Refer to the outline for key points, and reflect on your laboratory experience to answer this question.

LABORATORY EXERCISE 11
Radiographic Quality Assurance

1. D	5. C	9. C
2. D	6. A	10. C
3. D	7. C	
4. C	8. B	

LABORATORY EXERCISE 12
Radiographic Interpretation

1. C	5. D	9. D
2. A	6. C	10. D
3. C	7. D	
4. A	8. C	

LABORATORY EXERCISE 13
Supplemental Radiographic Techniques

1. B	5. A	9. B
2. C	6. C	10. A
3. A	7. C	
4. D	8. A	

LABORATORY EXERCISE 14
Panoramic Radiographic Technique

1.	A	4.	A	7.	A
2.	D	5.	B	8.	B
3.	B	6.	A	9.	D

10. Essay—See outline for key points to be included in this answer.

LABORATORY EXERCISE 15
Digital Radiography

1.	B	5.	C	9.	B
2.	D	6.	A	10.	A
3.	C	7.	C		
4.	B	8.	C		